Clinical Reasoning
in Patient Care

CLINICAL REASONING in PATIENT CARE

A. David Ginsburg

M.D. (Cape Town), F.C.P. (South Africa), M.R.C.P. (E), F.R.C.P. (C)

ASSOCIATE PROFESSOR OF MEDICINE
DIRECTOR CLINICAL SKILLS PROGRAM
DEPARTMENT OF MEDICINE, QUEEN'S UNIVERSITY,
KINGSTON, ONTARIO, CANADA

HARPER & ROW, PUBLISHERS
HAGERSTOWN

Cambridge
New York
Philadelphia
San Francisco

London
Mexico City
São Paulo
Sydney

1817

The author and publisher have exerted every effort to ensure that drug selection and dosage set forth in this text are in accord with current recommendations and practice at the time of publication. However, in view of ongoing research, changes in government regulations, and the constant flow of information relating to drug therapy and drug reactions, the reader is urged to check the package insert for each drug for any change in indications and dosage and for added warnings and precautions. This is particularly important when the recommended agent is a new or infrequently employed drug.

1 2 3 4 5

Library of Congress Cataloging in Publication Data

Ginsburg, A David
  Clinical reasoning in patient care.

  Bibliography
  Includes index.
  1. Diagnosis, Differential. 2. Medicine, Clinical
—Decision making. I. Title.
RC71.5.G56   616.07′5   80-10124
ISBN 0-06-140915-4

To my wife, Lynne,
and our children,
Neale, Daryl, and Alison

Contents

PREFACE   ix

ACKNOWLEDGMENTS   xi

1. PROBLEM FORMULATION AND CLINICAL REASONING   1

2. WEIGHT LOSS   7

3. HOARSENESS   23

4. DYSPNEA   30

5. CENTRAL CHEST PAIN   45

6. VOMITING   58

7. POLYURIA   74

8. JOINT PAIN   88

9. EASY BRUISING   102

10. HEADACHE   113

11. HYPERTENSION   126

12. HYPOTENSION 138

13. CLUBBING OF THE FINGERS 149

14. DULLNESS TO PERCUSSION 157

15. PLEURAL FLUID 163

16. JAUNDICE 176

17. SPLENOMEGALY 187

18. PERIPHERAL EDEMA 204

19. HEART FAILURE 211

20. PTOSIS 220

SUGGESTED READING 234

INDEX 235

Preface

The beginning medical student is taught a system for interviewing and examining a patient. The student is also taught the clinical manifestations of a large number of disease entities. Achieving an efficient interplay of these two bodies of knowledge often proves to be difficult for the beginning student. The purpose of this book is to try to illustrate how this may be achieved, and so facilitate clinical reasoning and problem solving.

The first chapter is concerned with an approach to the patient, and to problem formulation and analysis. The subsequent chapters are intended to illustrate how this approach to clinical problem solving may be applied, using as examples common clinical findings that may be encountered early in a student's career.

The format employed is intended to lead the reader through the steps of clinical reasoning. First, a problem is identified, sometimes in the form of a case history; next, questions are posed, just as might be done during rounds; the reader may attempt to find his own answers before referring to the answers in the text, which are presented last.

My intent has not been to be exhaustive but rather to try to emphasize priorities. Certainly there will be disagreement in many areas. My own bias as a hemato-oncologist will be clearly evident.

A. David Ginsburg

Acknowledgments

I acknowledge with much pleasure the contributions of many individuals to this book.

A "clinical approach" must reflect the cumulative effect of numerous influences. Several of my early teachers at the University of Cape Town played as important role in shaping my understanding of clinical reasoning. They include particularly Drs. Wilfred Baumann, Eugene Dowdle, Pat Smythe, Jannie Louw, Stuart Saunders, Geoff Thatcher, and Simmy Bank. I suspect that they are totally unaware of their impact, but I am nevertheless very pleased to acknowledge it.

Discussions with my wife, Dr. Lynne Ginsburg, have, over the years, molded my approach to patients, and she will recognize many of her ideas in these pages. For this, and for her support and encouragement during the preparation of this book, I am deeply grateful.

Several medical students have assisted me in the preparation of various aspects of the book, and I am happy to acknowledge the help of Colin McIver, Bill Cameron, Normal Hey, Stephen Archer, and Lois Champion.

A number of my colleagues in the Department of Medicine at Queen's University were kind enough to read sections of the original drafts and to make valuable suggestions. They include Drs. Tassos Anastassiades, Paul Armstrong, Charles Bird, Peter Galbraith, Aubrey Groll, Peter Munt, Joseph Pater, Jerry Simon, and Ronald Wigle. Drs. Larry Wilson and Vincent Young read the completed manuscript.

My secretary, Mrs. Margaret Axler, has spent endless hours typing and retyping the manuscript—always with good humor and patience. Her assistance has been invaluable.

It is a pleasure also to acknowledge the encouragement, enthusiasm, and editing wisdom of the staff at Harper & Row. They have all served to make this task both exciting and pleasurable.

CHAPTER 1

Problem Formulation and Clinical Reasoning

Much of the purpose of physical diagnosis courses is to provide the student with guidance in relating to patients, in structuring the interview, and in the categories of information that should be elicited from the interview, which include

1. Patient identification
2. The reason the patient sought medical help
3. The circumstances and details of the present illness
4. A screening survey composed of a review of the

   - Various body systems
   - Past history
   - Family history
   - Life situation
   - Medications and other forms of therapy
   - Alcohol, cigarette, and street-drug usage

The student is also taught how to perform a *physical examination* in a systematic and efficient manner.

A data base composed of symptoms and signs emerges from the history and physical examination. This information results in the perception of clinical problems which must be resolved.

To resolve a problem requires, initially, that the *cause* of the problem be defined as clearly as possible and that its potential *effects* be considered and assessed.

PROBLEM DEFINITION AND SELECTION

The first step in the clinical reasoning process is to decide which of the findings that have been or are being elicited are worth pursuing for their diagnostic and prognostic potential, and for possible therapeutic requirements. Thus it is very important not to be sidetracked into a premature analysis of the first symptom forthcoming, but rather to obtain an *overview* of a patient's symptoms and problems, listing them, if necessary, as the patient speaks, and selecting those that one wishes to evaluate.

This applies both to symptoms that the patient volunteers and to symptoms elicited in the course of the "screening survey"; to signs detected in the course of the routine physical examination; and to abnormal laboratory findings.

The appropriate selection of problems may be quite difficult, and constitutes a major component of "clinical judgement."

Some of the factors that contribute to the decision about the selection of a problem include

1. **The nature of the finding**

   • Central chest pain can never be overlooked.
   • An abdominal mass always demands an explanation.

2. **The severity of the finding**

   • A 20-lb weight loss is more likely to reflect significant disease than is a 2-lb weight loss.

3. **The course and duration of the finding**

   • A cough that has been progressive over 2 weeks is more likely to be significant than one that has been present, unchanged, for many years.

4. **The "clinical background"**

   • The development of even mild nausea and vomiting in a patient with known malignant disease would require very thorough attention.

5. **The extent to which the condition is bothering the patient**

The purpose of such problem definition is to serve as a guide to the subsequent approach to the patient. It is essential that problems be wisely formulated, at a level consistent with the student's knowledge and understanding, and *only* at a level that can be substantiated by the available evidence. Thus, if a patient were to complain of "dyspnea on effort," the problem would obviously be far better posed as one of "effort dyspnea" than one of "left-sided heart failure," until sufficient evidence were available to confirm the latter. Indeed much of the business of problem analysis is concerned with the gathering of evidence that will justify the more precise formulation of problems at ever higher levels of resolution, often in a stepwise fashion, until further resolution is impractical.

PROBLEM ANALYSIS

Once a problem has been formulated, it can then be analyzed—first, by considering two questions:

- What is its cause?
- What are its consequences?

CAUSE

When considering the cause of a particular problem, one usually begins by postulating several possibilities—i.e., by developing a *differential diagnosis.* In essence, this requires a reasonable knowledge base, and an awareness of what is probable, as opposed to what is possible.

Thus with regard to any problem, it is necessary to

1. **Know its common causes.**
2. **Be aware of the more probable causes in a particular patient, in view of that patient's known medical background.**
3. **Seek and be alert to clues in the history, physical examination, and routine laboratory examination of the patient that will enable one to develop a differential diagnosis appropriate to that patient**

In addition, it is essential to

4. **Be acutely aware of those causes—even if rare—that require urgent therapy, or that are amenable to specific treatment.**
5. **Have access to, or be able to develop, a comprehensive list of causes, when consideration of those suggested in the above categories fails to provide an acceptable solution.**

Once a number of possible causes have been identified, it is then
necessary to determine which is responsible. This next process
requires

1. *Knowledge* concerning the clinical and laboratory
   manifestations of the postulated disorders;
2. A reliable and efficient system for determining
   whether or not the anticipated manifestations are
   present—*the orderly, goal-directed history and physical examination;* and
3. Knowledge and judgment as to the *significance* of a
   finding in the context in which it is encountered.

Thus, once a problem has been formulated, its resolution
depends on the initial development of a reasoned differential
diagnosis. Evidence is then sought that will support or negate the
various probabilities, until one is confirmed, the particular
problem is solved, and a new one is posed.

By employing this approach of systematically postulating and
testing hypotheses, problems may be posed and resolved in a
stepwise and logical fashion, beginning at the student's level of
sophistication and progressing eventually to the highest point of
resolution that is reasonable. At each new step along the way a
differential diagnosis must be generated and explored, until
enough evidence is obtained to justify a new level of problem
formulation.

For example, if a patient were to complain of "fatigue," this
might well constitute one problem (among others) to be pursued.

Anemia, since it is a common cause of fatigue, would be one of
several probabilities to be considered. The possibility of anemia
might be supported by looking for, and detecting, pallor during
the directed physical examination, and then confirmed by
documenting a hemoglobin concentration of 4 gm/dl on specific
laboratory investigation.

One aspect of the problem, the cause for the patient's fatigue,
will have been resolved:

Fatigue

$\longrightarrow$ Anemia

The cause for the anemia must now be determined.

Several possible mechanisms for anemia exist. The possibility
of iron deficiency might be suggested in the course of the directed
physical examination by the presence of

- Koilonychia

- A blue discoloration of the sclerae
- A smooth tongue
- A blood film showing hypochromia and microcytosis

This could be confirmed in this patient by a bone-marrow aspirate showing an absence of iron stores.

The problem will have been resolved further:

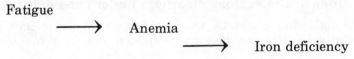

Fatigue

$\longrightarrow$ Anemia

$\longrightarrow$ Iron deficiency

A new problem will have been posed, but at a higher level of resolution.

The process of problem formulation and resolution might eventually progress to "carcinoma of the colon":

Fatigue

$\longrightarrow$ Anemia

$\longrightarrow$ Iron deficiency

$\longrightarrow$ Gastrointestinal blood loss

$\longrightarrow$ Carcinoma of the colon

It might now be reasonable to ask *why* the patient has a carcinoma of the colon, but this moves out of the realm of clinical medicine and into the sphere of research.

EFFECT

Just as it is important, when analyzing a problem, to attempt to establish its cause, so is it important to be aware of its possible consequences and to determine if they are present.

This will apply at each level of problem formulation and resolution. Thus, the potential effects of fatigue are quite different from those of anemia, or iron deficiency, or gastrointestinal bleeding, or carcinoma of the colon.

In order to recognize the effects of a problem, it is again necessary to

- Know their clinical manifestations, and
- Be able to detect them.

Again, the orderly history and physical examination constitutes an ideal means for this purpose.

Thus, the HISTORY and PHYSICAL serves several functions:

1. **It is the means for detecting many of the patient's problems;**
2. **It contributes to the development of the differential diagnosis;**
3. **It may be directed to seeking the specific manifestations of the various disorders under consideration.**

The following chapters are intended to illustrate how the principles described above may be applied in specific instances.

CHAPTER 2

Weight Loss

Loss of weight may present as a symptom noted by the patient, or as an objective sign detected by the physician. This is as important in the obese patient who loses weight as it is in the patient who was at, or below, optimum weight. Significant weight loss always warrants serious attention, since it is frequently the presenting symptom or sign of a major disease process.

What constitutes "significant" weight loss?

- If weight loss is a presenting complaint, this is obviously important.
- Weight loss greater than 10 percent of the initial weight is also clearly significant. Lesser degrees may be important and might need serial follow-up to detect a trend. Increasing loss of weight would be significant.
- Seasonal fluctuations in weight are much less likely to be meaningful.

Is weight loss always indicative of significant loss of tissue?

No. In many patients, especially hospitalized patients, weight loss reflects loss of edema fluid (and may hence be advantageous). Conversely, accumulation of edema fluid might mask the recognition of "true weight loss."

What symptoms or signs should alert you to the possibility of "weight loss" as a problem?

- The patient may volunteer that he has lost weight.

- In response to routine questioning in the "review of systems," the patient may recall losing weight.
- The patient may appear thin, emaciated, or cachectic.
- Physical examination may suggest that the patient's clothes are "too big" or baggy, or that skin turgor is diminished.

How may weight loss be confirmed?

- The patient may be aware of a change in collar size, dress size, waist measurement, etc.
- The patient may be aware of his previous weights, or maximum weight, which can be contrasted with his present weight.
- Weight loss may be documented on a bathroom scale (fraught with fallacies!).
- Most patients are weighed routinely when seen by a physician or admitted to the hospital. Comparison of present weight with such records will permit objective confirmation of weight loss.
- Prospective serial weighing will confirm progressive weight loss.

ILLUSTRATIVE CASE HISTORY

During your physical diagnosis course you are asked to evaluate a 48-year-old man who has been admitted to the hospital for investigation of weight loss.

He had been well 2 months previously when he began to notice increasing loss of weight. He had "always" weighed between 165 and 170 lbs. He now weighs 145 lbs.

What factors can result in weight loss?

- Diminished calorie (food) intake
- "Loss" of food, from persistent vomiting
- Impaired digestion or absorption of food (a malabsorption state)
- Increased need for, and utilization of calories, such as might occur in thyrotoxicosis
- "Loss" of calories, as in the glycosuria of diabetes mellitus

What are the more likely causes of weight loss in this North American middle-aged adult?

- Malignant disease
- Depression
- Diabetes mellitus
- Thyrotoxicosis
- A chronic infection
- A malabsorptive state

How might you reasonably begin to evaluate this patient?

First, with a **REVIEW OF SYMPTOMS** relevant to the GASTROINTESTINAL SYSTEM.

- *Dietary details* would be of paramount importance. The nature and amount of food eaten at breakfast, lunch, dinner, and at other times, should be determined. A *change in dietary habits* could be very significant:
  - A deliberate reduction in food intake, in an attempt to lose weight, would reduce the clinical significance of weight loss, although not uncommonly, successful dieting will coincide with the onset of significant disease.
  - A normal or increased appetite and dietary intake accompanying weight loss would be very suggestive of diabetes mellitus or thyrotoxicosis, but might also be compatible with malignant disease.
  - Conversely, anorexia, with a diminished dietary intake for this reason, would be suggestive of depression, infection, or malignant disease. (Other factors such as endogenous toxins—for example, uremia or liver failure; or exogenous toxins—drugs, poisons—might be responsible.)
  - Vomiting needs consideration, since the effects of a good diet could be vitiated by infrequent vomiting.
- A change in *bowel habit* or in the *character of the stool* might be a clue to a malabsorptive state. While the stool may be normal in these disorders, a history of diarrhea, or of the passage of loose, bulky, frothy, greasy, foul-smelling stools that are difficult to flush would be very suspicious.

On talking to your patient you learn that he has not been dieting. His appetite, however, has lessened, and he is not enjoying his food. His meals are smaller in quantity than previously. There has been no nausea or vomiting. He is somewhat constipated, but there is no other bowel abnormality.

What disorders would you now consider as likely to account for his weight loss?

- Depression
- Malignant disease
- Chronic infection

DEPRESSION

How might you pursue the possibility of a depressive illness in this patient?

An orderly **HISTORY** is, as always, a powerful investigative tool.

A **SYSTEMS REVIEW** should be pursued, with regard to

1. His Emotional Adjustments

- He may recognize and admit to feeling depressed, "low," or despondent, and to suicidal thoughts.
- He may have become irritable, with a deterioration in his family, social, and work relationships.
- His waking hours may be concerned with an "endless round-about" of painful thoughts and ideas of worthlessness and failure; and his attitudes toward the future may be very bleak.

2. His General Health

- There might be evidence of fatigue, listlessness, and lack of energy. These symptoms, in depression, will be present even on awakening. They may improve somewhat over the course of the day.
- Small tasks may seem to require great effort, so that he may complain of having little interest in performing his day-to-day activities.

3. His Habits

There may be evidence of

- *Insomnia.* He may have difficulty falling asleep, awaken frequently and early, and feel as if he had not slept at all. When he does sleep, his dreams may have a nightmarish quality.
- *Loss of libido* and/or impotence.

With regard to the **PAST HISTORY**, there may be a record of

- Depressive or manic illness
- Electroconvulsive therapy
- Antidepressant drug therapy
- Suicide attempts, or
- Admission to a psychiatric facility

With regard to the **FAMILY HISTORY**, there may be evidence of

- Depression, mania, or suicide
- Admission to a mental hospital, or
- The need for psychiatric care, in other family members

With regard to the **CURRENT LIFE SITUATION**

- There may be evidence of problems—domestic, occupational, or social—which may have precipitated a depressive illness (but which could also be consequent on it).
- He may have a lessened interest and participation in social activities.
- His alcohol intake may have increased significantly.

OBSERVATION of the patient may also be very useful:

- He may "look" depressed or sad, or may cry easily.
- There may be little or no spontaneous smiling.
- Speech and movements may be slow and laborious.
- His posture may be "slumped."

MALIGNANT DISEASE

How might you pursue the possibility of a malignant process in this patient?

The presence and site of a malignant process may quickly become obvious. However, an occult malignancy might well be responsible for the 20-lb weight loss in this man, and would require meticulous attention to detail for its detection.

Skillful utilization of the **HISTORY** and **PHYSICAL EXAMINATION** will often provide a precise guide to the necessary investigations and confirmatory diagnostic tests.

How might a carefully structured history and physical examination aid in localizing, or at least in furthering the suspicion, of malignant disease?

You might be able to elicit additional symptoms or signs resulting from the disease. These may arise from the manifestations of

- The primary tumor
- The regional spread of tumor
- Distant spread of tumor
- The development of paraneoplastic syndromes
- Other systemic symptoms

In considering a diagnosis of malignant disease, evidence that a patient is at increased risk for developing a particular malignancy might also have diagnostic value.

What are the more common tumors that should be considered?

In a man, these include

- Carcinoma of the
  - Lung
  - Colon
  - Prostate, or
  - Pancreas

In a female

- Carcinoma of the
  - Breast
  - Ovaries, or
  - Cervix

require specific attention.

- The leukemia/lymphoma group of malignancies is less common but should also be remembered.

What sites are commonly involved by metastic disease?

- Lymph nodes
- Liver
- Lungs and pleura
- Bones
- Brain

What are the more common paraneoplastic syndromes, and what is their significance?

None is especially common, but their detection in a patient whom you are investigating for weight loss would certainly heighten the possibility of malignant disease. The more common paraneoplastic syndromes include:

- Skin lesions
- Hematopoietic abnormalities
- Endocrine disorders
- Connective tissue disorders, and
- Neuromuscular disorders.

What are the "systemic" manifestations of malignant disease?

- Fever
- Sweating
- Chills
- Lassitude
- Fatigue
- Anorexia, and
- Weight loss

With these factors in mind, how might you structure the HISTORY in an attempt to detect and localize a malignancy?

A careful and detailed **REVIEW OF SYSTEMS** is the first requisite. With regard to

1. His General Health

- Unexplained, persistent, or recurrent *fever,* and fatigue and lassitude, are nonspecific symptoms that do, however, increase the probability of malignant disease. In contrast to its manifestations in the depressed patient, fatigue due to organic disease is *not* usually evident on awakening, but develops and progresses over the course of the day.

2. The Respiratory System

The recent development (or change in character) of

- Cough and sputum production
- Hemoptysis
- Dyspnea
- Chest pain
- Wheezing, and
- Hoarseness

might be indicative of either primary or metastatic involvement of the lungs and/or pleura.

3. The Gastrointestinal System

- *Anorexia, nausea, and vomiting* are fairly nonspecific symptoms, but might suggest a carcinoma of the stomach.
- *Dysphagia* is an important symptom of carcinoma of the esophagus, stomach, or bronchus.
- *Hematemesis* would suggest a carcinoma of the stomach.
- *Abdominal* pain or *discomfort* is a very significant symptom:
  - Carcinoma of the *pancreas* could present with epigastric or nonspecific pain.
  - Carcinoma of the *colon* might manifest with the colic of large bowel obstruction.
  - Hepatic metastases, especially if infarcted, might provoke right upper quadrant discomfort.
- A change in *bowel habit* would be highly indicative of gastrointestinal cancer, as would a change in the *character of the stools*—especially the passage of melena, fresh blood and/or mucus, or very pale stools.
- *Jaundice* might indicate a carcinoma of the head of the pancreas, or metastatic liver involvement.
- An *increase in abdominal girth* would suggest a large abdominal mass, significant hepatomegaly from metastatic disease, or the development of malignant ascites.

4. The Cardiovascular System

- *Deep vein thrombosis*—especially if recurrent and otherwise unexplained—would very much support the probability of malignant disease, as would *thrombophlebitis migrans.*
- *Swelling of the face and upper limbs* might be indicative of of malignant pericarditis and tamponade, or of superior vena caval obstruction.

5. The Genitourinary System

Symptoms might be due to a primary malignancy of the genitourinary tract, and might also be a consequence of metastatic disease causing obstruction, diminished bladder capacity, or vesicointestinal fistulae.

A detailed review of symptoms relevant to this system might thus be very useful:

- *Costovertebral angle pain* might reflect a renal tumor, or hydronephrosis due to ureteric obstruction by tumor.
- *Ureteric colic* might also reflect such obstruction.
- *Suprapubic discomfort,* or *pain,* would suggest urinary retention in a patient with prostatic cancer; cystitis consequent on prostatic cancer and obstruction; or a primary bladder cancer.
- A variety of *abnormal patterns of micturition* might also be indicative of malignant disease:
  - *Frequency* might indicate a space-occupying mass in the pelvis.
  - *Frequency* and *dysuria* would suggest an irritative lesion of the bladder.
  - *Obstructive symptoms:* difficulty in initiating micturition, hesitancy, interruption of the stream, or decreased size and force of the stream might indicate prostatic malignancy, as might *overflow incontinence.*
- *Hematuria* is a very significant symptom that would suggest malignancy anywhere in the genitourinary tract.
- *A testicular swelling* would be ominous.

6. The Musculoskeletal System

Symptoms usually result from distant spread of tumor, but might reflect a paraneoplastic syndrome, or regional spread.

- *Bone pain* is a very significant symptom in all of these regards.
- *Joint pain* or swelling might represent a paraneoplastic manifestation.

7. The Skin

- *Pruritus* might indicate a lymphoma.
- *A skin rash* could be a very significant sign of metastatic disease or of a variety of cutaneous paraneoplastic syndromes.

8. The Nervous System

A careful review of the symptoms pertaining to this system is very important:

- Loss of consciousness
- Convulsions
- Headache
- Disturbances of vision, speech, swallowing
- Weakness and muscle wasting
- Disturbance of balance and coordination
- Vertigo

are all symptoms which could reflect either metastatic disease or a paraneoplastic syndrome.

Had this been a female patient, careful additional inquiry into symptoms referable to the reproductive system would be mandatory. Thus, with regard to:

1. The Genital Tract

- Postmenopausal bleeding
- Contact bleeding following intercourse or douching, or
- A vaginal discharge

might all indicate malignant disease.

2. The Breast

A history of

- A breast lump
- Enlargement of a breast
- Shrinkage of a breast

- Itching, redness, or retraction of a nipple
- A nipple discharge

would all suggest breast cancer.

THE PAST HISTORY and A REVIEW OF THE PROBLEM LIST might yield very valuable information:

- Previous documentation of malignant disease, irrespective of the time interval;
- Previous surgery—especially abdominal or breast—if there were any doubt at all as to its basis; and
- Prior documentation of a "premalignant" disorder—*e.g.,* ulcerative colitis or intestinal polyposis

—must all enhance the probability that the patient now has active malignant disease.

- A history of recurrent infection of the respiratory or urinary tracts would be very suggestive of cancer in these sites, or of leukemia, lymphoma, or myeloma.
- Prior significant exposure to radiation would also enhance the suspicion of malignant disease.

THE FAMILY HISTORY. A few tumors have a definite familial incidence, with an apparent dominant inheritance pattern. Documentation of such tumors in close family members would therefore be of value for a specific patient.
These tumors include

- Multiple endocrine adenomatoses such as
  - ○ Pheochromocytoma
  - ○ Medullary thyroid carcinoma
  - ○ Islet cell tumors of the pancreas
- Polyposis coli and adenocarcinoma

Some of the more common tumors may also have increased familial incidence patterns and, again, a family history of such tumors would raise the suspicion of a similar tumor in the patient. Tumors with perhaps a three-fold incidence in immediate relatives include:

- Carcinoma of the breast, stomach, colon, prostate, or lung
- Melanoma

THE LIFE SITUATION. A variety of clues might stem from a consideration of this component of the history.

1. Geographic Factors

Certain tumors have a specific geographic preponderance. Thus:

- In a Japanese patient who is losing weight, carcinoma of the stomach would be especially suspect.
- In a Chinese—carcinoma of the nasopharynx.
- In an African—carcinoma of the esophagus or liver, or Burkitt's lymphoma.
- In an Egyptian—carcinoma of the bladder.

2. Occupational Factors

- Industrial exposure has been associated with certain malignancies. Thus, for example:
  - Miners exposed to radon, nickel, or silica would be at risk for carcinoma of the lung.
  - Dye and rubber industry workers are at risk for bladder cancer.
  - Asbestos workers would be at risk for carcinoma of the lung or a pleural mesothelioma.

USE OF ALCOHOL, CIGARETTES, AND DRUGS

- Cigarette smoking is classically associated with carcinoma of the lung, and perhaps also of the bladder.
- Excess alcohol consumption might be a clue to cancer of the mouth, pharynx, esophagus, or liver.

MEDICATIONS

- Prior exposure to alkylating agents and/or radiation therapy must raise the suspicion of malignant disease, especially leukemia.

What aspects of the PHYSICAL EXAMINATION would be important when considering malignant disease?

The especially significant features are listed in Table 2-1.

INFECTION

Any of a variety of infections might present with weight loss.

TABLE 2-1. PHYSICAL SIGNS OF POTENTIAL SIGNIFICANCE IN THE PATIENT WITH SUSPECTED MALIGNANT DISEASE

Source	Sign	Potential significance
General appearance	Chronic ill health Cachexia	Nonspecific, but suspicious
Mental status	Organic brain syndrome	Nonspecific, possibly suspicious
The hand	Clubbing of the fingers Nicotine staining Wasting of small muscles	Carcinoma of the lung
The skin	A variety of lesions	Metastatic disease Paraneoplastic syndromes
The head	Cranial nerve palsies	Metastatic disease
Fundus	Papilledema	Cerebral metastases
The eye	Proptosis Horner's syndrome	Metastatic disease—especially cancer of the breast, or lung, or a lymphoma
	Jaundice	Hepatic involvement by tumor Carcinoma of the pancreas
The face	Edema and suffusion	Superior vena caval obstruction; pericardial tamponade
	"Moon" facies	Ectopic ACTH production—a paraneoplastic disorder
The neck	Lymphadenopathy	Lymphoma Metastatic disease
	Distended veins	Superior vena caval obstruction; pericardial tamponade
	Hoarseness	Recurrent laryngeal nerve palsy due to tumor Superior vena caval obstruction
The thorax	Signs of consolidation, atelectasis, or effusion A localized wheeze	Primary or metastatic disease of the lung
The breasts and axillae	Mastectomy scar Breast lump Nipple changes	Cancer of the breast
	Axillary adenopathy	Cancer of the breast Lymphoma
Abdomen	Hepatomegaly Ascites	Metastatic disease
	Splenomegaly	Lymphoma
	Mass	Carcinoma
Rectum	Mass	Carcinoma of the rectum (if intrinsic) Pelvic organ malignancy Metastatic spread
	Prostatic irregularity	Carcinoma of the prostate
Scrotum	Testicular mass	Testicular carcinoma
Spine	Tenderness	Metastatic disease Myeloma
Extremities	Localizing CNS signs	Paraneoplastic syndromes Metastatic disease

Clues to the presence and site of an infectious process might be forthcoming from the **HISTORY**—particularly the **SYSTEMS REVIEW,** and a review of the **LIFE SITUATION.**

Tuberculosis and bacterial endocarditis are always worth specific consideration.

How might the SYSTEMS REVIEW contribute to the diagnosis?

With regard to

1. The Patient's General Health

2. The Respiratory System

Those symptoms that would suggest malignant disease might equally suggest an infectious process.

3. The Gastrointestinal Tract

- Diarrhea would suggest an intestinal infection.

4. The Genitourinary Tract

- Frequency and dysuria would be very suggestive of infection.

How might a review of the LIFE SITUATION contribute?

A history of travel to, or origin in, exotic countries would certainly suggest an infection endemic to those areas.

What aspects in the history would increase the suspicion of TUBERCULOSIS in this patient?

THE REVIEW OF SYSTEMS might reveal, with regard to the patient's

1. General Health

- Late afternoon fever
- Night sweats
- Fatigue and lassitude

2. Respiratory System

- A dry or productive cough

- Hemoptysis
- Dyspnea, and/or
- A persistent chest infection, or "cold"

There might be, with regard to the

PAST HISTORY

- Prior documentation of tuberculosis
- Recurrent chest infections

FAMILY HISTORY

- Documentation of tuberculosis in other family members

LIFE SITUATION

- Contact with tuberculous subjects at home or work
- Origin in, or travel to, endemic areas

What aspects in the history would suggest BACTERIAL ENDO-CARDITIS?

In addition to nonspecific symptoms of infection, if there were, with regard to the **PAST HISTORY**

- Prior documentation of rheumatic fever or valvular heart disease, or
- A history of recent dental work or genitourinary investigation

—this would be very suspicious.

What physical findings would enhance the suspicion of bacterial endocarditis?

These are reviewed in the chapter on Finger Clubbing.

From the history and physical examination you learn that your patient has "always" had a smoker's cough, but that this has perhaps worsened recently. There was some blood-streaking of the sputum on one occasion 3 weeks previously.

He has smoked one package of cigarettes a day for 30 years.

He has slight but definite finger clubbing, but no other abnormal findings on physical examination.

What do these features suggest?

That he has carcinoma of the lung.

How will you try to confirm this?

Sophisticated, goal-directed laboratory tests may now reasonably be instituted.

- Chest radiography
- Hilar tomography
- Cytological evaluation of the sputum
- Bronchoscopy

may all be helpful.

Sputum cytology shows evidence of a squamous cell carcinoma, and bronchoscopy and biopsy confirm this diagnosis.

How should you proceed?

The questions to be posed now are:

- What is the appropriate management for this patient?
- What is his prognosis?

Answers will depend upon determining

- The extent of the carcinoma—locally, regionally, and distantly
- His general condition
- His pulmonary function status
- His family, occupational, and financial circumstances

CHAPTER 3

Hoarseness

A 44-year-old male patient is noted to be "hoarse"—his voice has an unusually low pitch, with a rough quality, when you see him at an outpatient clinic.

How much attention should you afford this observation?

While hoarseness is common, and usually benign, it always warrants an explanation.

What is the clinical significance of hoarseness?

- It indicates laryngeal dysfunction, which implies local pathology, and may reflect a systemic disease process.
- It may be uncomfortable for, or even distressing to, the patient.
- It may sometimes precede, or be associated with laryngeal obstruction.

What are the common causes for hoarseness?

- An acute upper respiratory tract infection
- Acute or chronic vocal abuse
- Vocal cord nodes or polyps

What significant systemic diseases may manifest with hoarseness?

- Myxedema
- Carcinoma—of the lung, and breast (in a female), particularly

23

What other important causes for hoarseness should be considered?

1. Intrinsic Laryngeal Pathology

- Foreign body
- Laryngitis—
  - ○ Fungal
  - ○ Tuberculous, or
  - ○ Syphylitic
- Carcinoma of the larynx

2. Neurologic Dysfunction

- Recurrent laryngeal nerve palsies

With this knowledge of possible causes, how might you try to establish the diagnosis in your patient?

A review of the **PROBLEM LIST** might reveal documentation of disorders that would render one or another of these causes more likely. Thus:

- In the immediately postoperative patient, hoarseness usually results from endotracheal intubation and the associated laryngeal irritation and inflammatory response.
- Following cervical surgery, and especially thyroid surgery, larnygeal nerve irritation (or even section?) would need to be considered.
- In a patient with known malignant disease
  - ○ Recurrent laryngeal nerve involvement by tumor
  - ○ The local effects of radiotherapy
  - ○ A monilial infection of the larynx resulting from immunosuppressive therapy.
  - ○ The virilizing effects of androgenic steroid therapy (in a female)

—would all need consideration.

- An alcoholic subject would be especially at risk for
  - ○ Nonspecific chronic laryngitis
  - ○ Tuberculosis of the larynx
  - ○ Syphilis of the larynx, or
  - ○ Carcinoma of the larynx

In the absence of such clues from the problem list, the routine **HISTORY** will usually permit ready confirmation of one of the common causes or provide a clue to the possibility of other disorders. Thus the history relevant to the hoarseness may reveal

- A *sudden onset*—suggestive of aspiration of a foreign body. (This would, however, be very unlikely to present as an incidental finding in an outpatient setting!)
- A *rapid onset* and *short duration,* of several days at the most, suggestive of an upper respiratory infection, acute vocal abuse, or neurologic disease
- A more *gradual onset,* with a more *prolonged course,* suggestive of
  - Chronic vocal abuse
  - Vocal cord nodes or polyps
  - Chronic laryngitis
  - Carcinoma of the larynx, or
  - Neurologic disease

The **REVIEW OF SYSTEMS** might reveal, with regard to

1. The Patient's General Health

- Fever—suggestive of an upper respiratory tract infection

2. The Respiratory System. Preceding or associated

- Sore throat
- Rhinorrhea
- Catarrh
- Cough, and/or the
- Central burning chest pain of tracheitis

—all suggestive of an acute infective process.

Review of the **PAST HISTORY** might reveal

- A previous diagnosis of vocal cord nodes
- A propensity to laryngitis, with previous upper respiratory tract infections
- Thyroid or parathyroid surgery; hence the potential for damage to the recurrent laryngeal nerve

Review of the **LIFE SITUATION** might reveal

- Recent, acute voice abuse from

○ Vigorous vocal participation in a sporting event or party, etc.

○ Inhalation of irritant gases

• Evidence for chronic voice abuse. Occupational factors such as

○ Auctioneering

○ Public speaking

○ Singing (badly), or

○ A dust-laden work environment

—might be important in this regard.

How might the PHYSICAL EXAMINATION contribute to the diagnosis?

With regard to

1. The General Appearance

• The features of a "cold" might be obvious.

2. The Head

• Redness and swelling of the eardrum, nasal mucous membrane, pharynx, and tonsils

• A nasal discharge

• A posterior pharyngeal "drip"

—would all be essentially confirmatory of an upper airway infection.

• A tonsillar or pharyngeal membrane should at least raise the suspicion of diphtheria.

• A swollen and inflamed epiglottis would suggest potentially lethal laryngotracheobronchitis

3. The Neck

• Upper cervical adenopathy would be supportive of a diagnosis of an upper respiratory tract infection, and if severe, of diphtheria.

On further evaluation of your patient, it is evident that his voice has been deepening over several weeks—in the absence of any precipitating or predisposing factors.

With an inspirational flash, you wonder if he could be myxedematous!

How might you pursue this possibility further, utilizing the HISTORY?

THE REVIEW OF SYSTEMS might reveal, with regard to

1. **General Health**
   - Weight gain
   - Increased sensitivity to cold
   - Easy fatigability
   - Weakness and lassitude

2. **The Gastrointestinal System**
   - Anorexia
   - Constipation

3. **The Cardiovascular System**
   - Chest pain of angina pectoris
   - Dyspnea on effort

4. **The Genitourinary System**
   - Loss of libido
   - (Increased menstrual blood loss)

5. **The Musculoskeletal System**
   - Vague muscle pains
   - "Heaviness" of the limbs

6. **The Nervous System**
   - Reduced mental functioning
   - Depression
   - Paresthesias in the median nerve distribution

7. **The Skin**
   - A change in the texture of the skin and hair
   - Loss of hair
   - An altered facial appearance

A review of the **PAST HISTORY** or **PROBLEM LIST** might reveal

- Previous documentation of thyrotoxicosis or other thyroid disease

- Treatment with radioactive iodine or thyroid suppressive drugs
- Previous thyroid surgery
- Previous documentation of hypothyroidism!
- Previous documentation of
  - Pernicious anemia
  - Rheumatoid arthritis
  - Addison's disease
  - Diabetes, or
  - Idiopathic thrombocytopenia

—disorders associated with an increased incidence of hypo-thyroidism.

What of the PHYSICAL EXAMINATION?

With regard to

1. The General Appearance

- The myxedematous patient is often slow of thought, speech, and movement.
- She is usually obese.

2. The Mental Status

- The memory is often poor.
- Apathy, drowsiness, and depression may be evident.

3. The Vital Signs

- Bradycardia and hypothermia may be evident.

4. The Head

- There is often a characteristic facies. The face may be pale and puffy, with thickening of the skin of the eyelids and cheeks, and with thickening of the lips and tongue.
- The hair may be coarse and lusterless, with some balding, and may be "difficult to manage." There may be loss of the outer eyebrows.

5. The Neck

- The thyroid may be impalpable, or enlarged, firm, and non-tender.

6. The Skin

- Thickening
- Roughening
- Dryness
- Coldness
- Bruising, and a
- Yellowish pigmentation

—may all be evident

7. **The Cardiovascular System.** There may be evidence of a pericardial effusion or of congestive cardiac failure (see chapter on Peripheral Edema).

8. **The Nervous System.** The reflexes may be virtually pathognomonic, with marked slowing of the recovery phase of the reflex.

To your chagrin, you are unable to confirm this hypothesis, even with appropriate laboratory studies.

How should you proceed?

To tomography of the larynx; and to indirect laryngoscopy, if you are competent in this regard; or by referring the patient to an otorhinolaryngologist.

What might be learned from indirect laryngoscopy?

The vocal cords can be inspected. There might be evidence of

- Acute swelling and inflammation
- Thickening of the cords
- Symmetric pearly nodes
- A foreign body
- Other lesions
- An abnormal position and abnormal movement of the cords with phonation, indicative of a nerve palsy.

CHAPTER 4

Dyspnea

A complaint of "shortness of breath" is frequently encountered in clinical practice. It is an important symptom, since it is often the first, or major, clue to a significant underlying disease process. Furthermore, this symptom can prove severely incapacitating, and produce a disruption of the patient's lifestyle.

Dyspnea may develop acutely and be evident at rest. It may also manifest as a more chronic process, occurring only with exercise or effort. The causes for dyspnea tend to be different under these circumstances, although considerable overlap exists.

ACUTE DYSPNEA

On your first night "on call" as an intern in the hematology department, you are asked by the nurse in charge to see a 24-year-old female patient with acute leukemia who has become increasingly short of breath.

What causes for this particular patient's dyspnea should reasonably come to mind as you quickly dress and rush to the floor?

1. Those conditions that could be responsible for the rapid development of dyspnea, and would require

- *Emergency* therapy
  - A tension pneumothorax
  - Upper airway obstruction

- *Urgent treatment*
  - Pulmonary edema
  - Pulmonary embolism
  - Fulminating bacterial infection
  - Acute asthma
  - Significant atelectasis

2. Those conditions that are most probable in patients with acute leukemia:

- Bacterial infection
- Other infections
- Pulmonary hemorrhage

3. Those conditions to which this patient with acute leukemia would be prone:

- Disease of the major airways
  - Aspiration of vomitus or other foreign material
  - Obstruction by enlarged lymph nodes.
- Disease of the pulmonary parenchyma
  - *Infection*—especially bacterial, but also viral, fungal, or parasitic
  - Drug-induced pneumonitis
  - Pulmonary hemorrhage
  - Pulmonary edema
  - Adult respiratory distress syndrome
  - Leukemic infiltrates
  - Pulmonary atelectasis
- Disease of the pulmonary vessels
  - Pulmonary embolism
  - Leukostasis
- Disease of the pleura
  - Pleural effusion or empyema
  - Pneumothorax
- Disease of the heart
  - Pericardial hemorrhage or tamponade
  - Infiltration of the myocardium by leukemic cells
  - Damage to the myocardium by drugs
- Anxiety

What circumstances would suggest that urgent assessment is indicated?

- An aura of panic as you arrive on the floor (guaranteed to disrupt your already dubious equanimity).
- A patient who is obviously restless and distressed, or who is unconscious.
- A patient who is cyanosed.
- Lung biopsy, pleural aspiration, or other pulmonary procedures having been done that day.
- Onset of dyspnea while eating, or following vomiting.

How would you proceed in these circumstances?

Directly to the physical examination, looking specifically for signs of

- A tension pneumothorax, and
- Upper airway obstruction

What are the signs of a tension pneumothorax?

- On inspection of the chest
  - Tachypnea
  - Diminished respiratory excursion on the side with the pneumothorax
  - Deviation of the apex beat and trachea to the opposite side
- On palpation
  - Confirmation of these observations
- On percussion
  - A hyperresonant percussion note over the abnormal side
- On auscultation
  - Absent, or a markedly diminished intensity of breath sounds
  - Absent or diminished vocal resonance

—on the abnormal side.

If these signs were apparent in a distressed patient, immediate therapy would be indicated. (*What would you do?*)

What are the signs of upper airway obstruction?

- General *observation,* and *inspection* of the chest may reveal
  - Tachypnea
  - Stridor
  - Indrawing of the suprasternal notch, intercostal spaces, and subcostal areas on inspiration.
  - Use of accessory muscles of respiration
- *Palpation* of the trachea may reveal a tracheal tug.
- *Auscultation* may be very noisy because of coarse crackles and inspiratory wheezes, and the breath sounds may be diminished in intensity.

If acute and severe large-airway obstruction were diagnosed, immediate therapy would again be indicated. (*What would you do?*)

Once you have determined that you are not dealing with an emergency situation, how would you now logically attempt to determine the cause for the patient's dyspnea? How might the HISTORY assist you?

A more detailed analysis concerning the **ONSET** and **COURSE** of the dyspnea might be useful:

- A sudden onset would suggest
  - Pulmonary embolism
  - A pneumothorax
  - Aspiration
- A rapid onset would suggest
  - Pulmonary edema
  - Pulmonary hemorrhage
  - A fulminating infection
- Progression over a few days would suggest
  - Pulmonary infection
  - A pleural effusion
  - Heart disease

THE REVIEW OF SYSTEMS might reveal, with regard to the patient's

1. General Health

- Fever, suggestive of an infective process

2. Respiratory System

- Pleuritic pain, suggestive of
  - Infection
  - Pulmonary embolism and infarction
  - A pneumothorax, or
  - A pleural effusion
- Wheezing, suggestive of
  - Asthma
  - Pulmonary embolism
  - Infection

3. Cardiovascular System

- Pain or swelling in a leg, indicative of deep vein thrombosis, and hence suggestive of
  - Pulmonary embolism

4. Central Nervous System

- Drowsiness or stupor *preceding* the dyspnea, and hence suggestive of
  - Aspiration
- Anxiety, possibly indicative of a
  - Psychogenic basis for the dyspnea

A REVIEW OF THE PROBLEM LIST, especially as it pertains to the **status of the leukemia,** might be very useful:

- A very low leukocyte count would be highly suggestive of pulmonary infection, while a very high count might indicate leukostasis.
- A low platelet count, or evidence of disseminated intravascular coagulation, would be compatible with pulmonary hemorrhage, or the adult respiratory distress syndrome.
- Severe anemia might be at least partially contributory to the dyspnea, although dyspnea at rest is unusual in this circumstance.

A REVIEW OF THE PROBLEM LIST relevant to the **investigation and management of the leukemia** might also be useful:

- A recent lung biopsy, or pleural aspiration, would render a pneumothorax very likely.

- Blood transfusion, platelet transfusion, and intravenous fluid therapy might all be responsible for pulmonary edema, especially if there were a coexisting degree of renal failure or cardiac disease.
- Chemotherapy has been claimed to precipitate intravascular coagulation, the adult respiratory distress syndrome, and leukostasis.
- Chemotherapy can also be responsible for a drug-induced pneumonitis.

A PAST HISTORY or FAMILY HISTORY of asthma would obviously be important.

How might the PHYSICAL EXAMINATION be of diagnostic assistance?

An orderly physical examination is indicated, looking specifically for evidence of those disorders that you consider likely in this patient. This might reveal, with regard to

1. The General Appearance of the Patient

- An acutely ill patient in some distress—a situation that demands prompt action, but provides little of differential-diagnostic value.

2. The Vital Signs

- Fever, suggestive of a pneumonic illness
- Tachycardia and tachypnea, which also have little differential-diagnostic significance
- Pulsus paradoxus, which, in the presence of respiratory distress, also loses its diagnostic value; and/or
- Hypotension, suggestive of
  - Pulmonary embolism
  - A tension pneumothorax, or
  - Bacterial pneumonia and septicemia

3. The Appearance of the Sputum

- Any sputum production (especially if purulent), which would suggest pulmonary infection.
- Frankly bloody sputum, which would suggest
  - Pulmonary hemorrhage
  - Embolism and infarction

4. The Head

- Cyanosis, indicative of a serious respiratory problem, and suggestive of
  - A tension pneumothorax
  - Airway obstruction
  - Pulmonary embolism, and possibly
  - Severe infection

5. The Neck

- Elevation of the jugular venous pressure, suggestive of
  - Cardiac failure
  - Cardiac tamponade, and
  - Pulmonary embolism
- Prominent "a" waves, suggestive of
  - Pulmonary embolism
- Kussmaul's sign and a steep "y" descent, suggestive of cardiac tamponade

With regard to the more specific examination of the THORAX, how might INSPECTION and PALPATION help explain the dyspnea?

There may be evidence of

- Diminished respiratory excursion on one side of the chest, suggestive of a
  - Pneumonia
  - Atelectasis
  - Pneumothorax, or
  - Pleural effusion on that side
- Mediastinal shift, suggestive of a
  - Pleural effusion
  - Pneumothorax, or
  - Atelectasis

How might PERCUSSION help?

- A localized area of dullness to percussion would suggest
  - Pneumonic consolidation
  - Atelectasis

- "Stony dullness" would suggest
  - A pleural effusion
- Hyperresonance over one lung field would suggest
  - A pneumothorax

What might you learn from AUSCULTATION of the chest?

The **intensity** of the breath sounds might be diminished, suggestive of

- A pleural effusion
- A pneumothorax, or
- Significant atelectasis

Bronchial breathing might be evident, suggestive of

- Pneumonic consolidation

Additional sounds might be audible:

- Localized crackles, suggestive of
  - Consolidation
  - Atelectasis
- Diffuse crackles or basal crackles would suggest
  - Pulmonary edema
  - A pulmonary infiltrate
- Diffuse, high-pitched expiratory wheezing would suggest
  - Asthma
- A pleural friction rub would suggest
  - Consolidation and underlying pleurisy
  - Pulmonary embolism and infarction

What might you learn from the remainder of the PHYSICAL EXAMINATION?

Examination might reveal, with regard to

1. The Precordium

- Displacement of the apex beat. If this were not due to a mediastinal shift, it might imply left ventricular dilatation, and cardiac failure would be suspect.

- A prominent right-ventricular lift, suggestive of pulmonary embolism.
- Inability to palpate the apex beat, possibly indicative of pericardial fluid accumulation.
- A gallop rhythm, suggestive of cardiac failure or pulmonary embolism.
- A loud P2, suggestive of pulmonary embolism.

2. **The Abdomen**

- Hepatomegaly, suggestive of cardiac failure or tamponade, but also wholly explicable on the basis of the primary leukemic process.

3. **The Extremities**

- A tender and/or swollen limb, suggestive of pulmonary embolism resulting from deep vein thrombosis
- Edema, suggestive of
  o Cardiac failure or
  o Tamponade
- Petechiae or bruising, indicative of a bleeding tendency, hence suggestive of pulmonary hemorrhage

How should you proceed?

Throughout the "goal-directed" screening survey you have been looking for leads to more specific diagnostic entities. Thus, when a "lead" *is* obtained, it should obviously be fully explored, and further evidence should be sought in support of the diagnosis which it suggests.

Upon further evaluation of this patient, you learn that the dyspnea was of fairly sudden onset, and that there is associated pleuritic chest pain.

What is the differential diagnosis now?

- Pulmonary embolism
- Pneumonia

It is thus very reasonable to reevaluate your findings, or, if necessary, to reexamine the patient, looking for those features that will enable you to differentiate between these two disorders (see these subjects in Chaps. 5 and 14).

Both of these diagnoses remain highly probable, even in the absence of confirmatory or discriminatory findings. Laboratory investigations will need careful consideration.

What laboratory tests might contribute to confirmation of:

An infection?

- Chest radiographs
- Sputum morphology and cultures
- Blood cultures

Decisions will be necessary as to

- Transtracheal aspiration
- Open lung biopsy
- Treatment

Pulmonary embolism?

- Chest radiographs
- Lung scans
- Blood gas analyses

Decisions will be necessary as to

- Pulmonary angiography
- Treatment

DYSPNEA ON EXERTION

While working as an intern in the cardiology department, you see a 56-year-old woman who has been referred to the outpatient clinic because of the recent onset (within the past 2 months) of dyspnea on effort. She must stop and rest at least once while climbing the stairs to her second-floor apartment. Six months previously this was not necessary. More recently she has had to rest while making her bed; mopping the kitchen floor is a problem because of the dyspnea which it engenders. A carcinoma of the breast had been diagnosed 2 years previously.

TABLE 4-1. "SPECIFIC" PHYSICAL EXAMINATION IN A PATIENT WITH EFFORT DYSPNEA AND PREVIOUSLY DOCUMENTED BREAST CANCER

Source	Sign	Potential significance
General appearance	*Respiratory distress* Breathing with difficulty Use of accessory muscles Pursed-lip breathing Grunting	Respiratory disease, especially chronic obstructive pulmonary disease
Vital signs	Hypertension Pulsus paradoxus	Heart failure Pericardial tamponade Constrictive pericarditis COPD
The head	Pallor Cyanosis	Anemia Significant lung disease
The neck	Elevated jugular venous pressure	Heart failure Tamponade Constrictive pericarditis Superior vena caval obstruction
	+Absence of venous pulsation	Superior vena caval obstruction
	+Kussmal's sign and "steep y descent"	Tamponade or constrictive pericarditis
	+Prominent "a" waves	Pulmonary embolism
The thorax		
INSPECTION	Deformities Barrel-shaped chest Kyphosis	COPD Restrictive lung disease consequent possibly on spinal metastases and vertebral collapse
	Diminished respiratory excursion —bilateral, with characteristic pattern —unilateral	COPD Pleural effusion Atelectasis
	Asymmetry of the chest	Effusion Atelectasis (of some duration)
	Deviation of the apex beat or trachea	Effusion Atelectasis Pulmonary fibrosis Kyphoscoliosis
PALPATION	Confirmation, or initial detection, of above signs	Same diagnostic implications
	Diminished vocal fremitus —unilateral	Effusion Atelectasis
	—diffuse	COPD

(continued)

TABLE 4-1. "SPECIFIC" PHYSICAL EXAMINATION IN A PATIENT WITH EFFORT DYSPNEA AND PREVIOUSLY DOCUMENTED BREAST CANCER (*Continued*)

Source	Sign	Potential significance
PERCUSSION	Diminished cardiac and liver dullness	COPD
	Localized area of dullness to percussion	Effusion Atelectasis Pulmonary embolism and infarction An elevated hemidiaphragm due to phrenic nerve involvement by tumor or to subdiaphragmatic pathology
AUSCULTA-TION	Diffuse diminution in the intensity of the breath sounds	COPD
	Localized area of decreased intensity	Effusion Atelectasis Elevation of diaphragm
	A friction rub	Malignant involvement of the pleura Pulmonary embolism
	Bilateral basal crackles	Heart failure Pneumonitis
	Localized area of crackles	Atelectasis Pulmonary embolism
The precordium		
INSPECTION	Displacement of the apex beat	Effusion Atelectasis Fibrosis (localized area) Kyphoscoliosis Heart disease
PALPATION	Confirmation of inspection	
	Right ventricular lift	Pulmonary embolism
	Palpable P2	COPD
	Impalpable apex beat	Pericardial tamponade Constrictive pericarditis
AUSCULTA-TION	Diminished intensity of the heart sounds	Tamponade Constrictive pericarditis COPD
	A loud P2	Pulmonary embolism COPD
	A gallop rhythm	Heart failure Pulmonary embolism
The abdomen	Hepatomegaly	Metastatic breast cancer Heart failure Tamponade Constrictive pericarditis COPD (liver displaced, not enlarged)

(continued)

41

TABLE 4-1. "SPECIFIC" PHYSICAL EXAMINATION IN A PATIENT
WITH EFFORT DYSPNEA AND PREVIOUSLY DOCUMENTED
BREAST CANCER (Continued)

Source	Sign	Potential significance
	Ascites	Metastatic disease Heart disease Heart failure Tamponade Constrictive pericarditis
The extremities	Unilateral edema and/ or tenderness of a lower limb	Deep vein thrombosis and pulmonary embolism
	Bilateral edema	Heart failure Cor pulmonale Tamponade Constrictive pericarditis

What disorders are especially liable to be responsible for effort dyspnea in this patient with known breast cancer?

- *Lung disease,* especially:
    - A pleural effusion
    - Pulmonary atelectasis
    - Lymphangitic carcinomatosis
    - Pneumonitis, resulting from either chemotherapy or radiotherapy
    - Recurrent pulmonary emboli
- *Heart disease,* especially:
    - Cardiac failure, resulting from chemotherapy, radiation therapy, or estrogen or prednisone administration
    - Cardiac tamponade, resulting from either malignant pericarditis or radiation-induced pericarditis
- *Severe anemia,* resulting from a variety of possible mechanisms in this patient
- *Anxiety*

Ischemic heart disease and chronic obstructive pulmonary disease (COPD) are sufficiently common to warrant specific consideration in any patient with effort dyspnea.

What features in the history might be of differential diagnostic value?

A **REVIEW OF SYMPTOMS** might reveal, in

1. The Cardiovascular System

- *Orthopnea,* indicative of left heart failure,or possibly COPD.
- *Paroxysmal nocturnal dyspnea,* which would also be very suggestive of heart failure, but which would need to be differentiated from bronchial asthma, or pulmonary embolism, and from the acute effects of sputum accumulation. If cough were a significant component of such episodes, this would mitigate against heart failure.
- *Ankle swelling,* which would certainly suggest cardiac disease, but which could be consequent on cor pulmonale, and which could be a clue to deep vein thrombosis, with recurrent pulmonary embolism being responsible for the effort dyspnea; or which could be due to severe anemia.
- *Central chest pain,* indicative of angina pectoris, and favoring ischemic heart disease as the cause of the dyspnea, but which could also be the result of anemia, pulmonary embolism, pericarditis, or possibly anxiety.

2. The Respiratory System

- Cough
- Sputum production
- Wheezing
- Hemoptysis
- Pleuritic chest pain

—all of which would favor the presence of lung disease to account for effort dyspnea.

Consideration of the **PAST HISTORY OR PROBLEM LIST** might reveal a previous diagnosis of heart disease, respiratory disease, anemia, or psychoneurotic illness—with the obvious implications; or of diseases likely to be complicated by disorders of these systems—*e.g.,* deep vein thrombosis and pulmonary embolism; systemic lupus erythematosus and pleural effusion; hypertension and left heart failure.

A consideration of the **FAMILY HISTORY** might reveal

- A familial incidence of chronic lung disease, or of heart disease

While this would suggest similar disease in the patient, it could also be the basis for an anxiety state.

Consideration of the **LIFE SITUATION** might reveal

- Situations where exposure to dusts might have occurred, suggestive of a pneumoconiosis
- Circumstances likely to precipitate anxiety—domestic, financial or occupational concerns, or the malignancy per se
- Evidence of an unstable personality

Review of the patient's **USE OF ALCOHOL, CIGARETTES, OR DRUGS** might reveal evidence of

- A significant smoking history, suggestive of chronic respiratory disease, or of ischemic heart disease
- Alcohol excesses, possibly suggestive of an alcoholic cardiomyopathy and heart failure

The **MEDICATION AND TREATMENT HISTORY** might be very significant:

- The use and extent of radiotherapy might be a clue to radiation pneumonitis, or carditis.
- Drug therapy is important, relevant to drug administration that may be associated with a pneumonitis—*e.g.,* bleomycin, busulfan; or cardiac failure—*e.g.,* adriamycin, or estrogens.

What signs will you look for specifically in the orderly PHYSICAL EXAMINATION in order to try to determine more precisely the cause for the patient's dyspnea?

The signs are listed in Table 4-1, together with their potential clinical significance.

What investigations are indicated?

- Hemoglobin concentration
- Chest radiograph
- Selected pulmonary function studies
- Electrocardiogram
- Arterial blood gas analyses

What further investigations are indicated?

A thoughtful examination might in itself resolve the cause for this patient's dyspnea—or certainly serve to exclude a number of options. Judicious tests might then be selected to confirm the clinical impression (if necessary), or further consider remaining possibilities.

CHAPTER 5

Central Chest Pain

During your rotation in the emergency department, a 58-year-old man is brought in, by his more than anxious family, with a 1-hour history of central chest pain of sudden onset. The resident on duty suggests that you see and assess him.

How might you begin to approach this problem?

Retrosternal pain or discomfort may indicate a life-threatening illness. Conversely, even excruciating pain in this region may be merely the result of dyspepsia and have no major clinical significance.

Because of the prevalence and potentially serious and urgent consequences of myocardial infarction, it would be wise to approach this patient from the viewpoint of whether he does or does not have a myocardial infarction and, more particularly, whether any of the urgent consequences *requiring immediate therapy* is evident.

What are the serious early complications of an acute myocardial infarction?

These include:

- Cardiac arrhythmias
- Hypotension and shock
- Left heart failure and pulmonary edema
- Ruptured papillary muscles
- Interventricular septal defect

How may these be assessed from the HISTORY?

Complaints of severe dyspnea and/or cough occurring with, or since, the onset of the pain would suggest acute left heart failure—possibly resulting from a ruptured papillary muscle or a ventricular septal defect.

Syncope would suggest significant hypotension and/or an arrhythmia.

In the present context these symptoms could also indicate a massive pulmonary embolism.

How may these complications be assessed from a very specific PHYSICAL EXAMINATION?

The *pulse rate* might be very slow, very fast, or irregular, indicating an arrhythmia.

The *pulse volume* might be significantly diminished, suggesting hypotension.

The *blood pressure* might be significantly reduced.

Auscultation of *the lungs* might reveal widespread crackles, suggestive of pulmonary edema; auscultation of the *precordium* might reveal a systolic murmur, suggesting papillary muscle dysfunction or rupture, or a ventricular septal defect.

How may they be assessed from laboratory studies?

An electrocardiogram might confirm acute myocardial injury and help to define the nature of a clinically detectable arrhythmia.

If any of these serious complications were evident, how should you proceed?

Management of the complications per se would be critical at this point, and you would need expert assistance—without delay.

In the absence of these complications, how might you reasonably proceed?

The possibility of acute myocardial infarction remains paramount, even in the absence of a characteristic ECG; and you should now try to decide, on the basis of a history, physical examination, and laboratory studies, if this is indeed the case.

How may the HISTORY contribute to this decision?

THE DESCRIPTION OF THE PAIN may be useful. This is often characteristic, including, as regards its

- Onset, course and duration
  - A sudden onset, persistent over several hours
- Site and radiation
  - A retrosternal site, with radiation often to the arms and/or sometimes to the jaw, neck, back, and abdomen
- Character and severity
  - A "squeezing" or "pressing" quality of pain that is usually extremely severe
- Aggravating (or precipitating) and relieving factors
  - A lack of any specific precipitating factors, with no evident relieving factors other than powerful analgesic administration. In particular, there is no relief from nitroglycerin.
- Associated factors
  - The presence of nausea and vomiting, dyspnea, "dizziness," syncope, and sweating

In this regard, it must be remembered that severe dyspnea might also indicate pulmonary embolism, while nausea, belching and vomiting might indicate gastrointestinal tract disease.

Dizziness and syncope could also reflect pulmonary embolism.

Could the patient still have an infarction even if he does not have so classical a history?

Yes. The pain might be gradual in onset; it might be felt only in the areas of radiation, and not centrally at all; the quality might vary considerably, and it need not be severe. In some instances it may even be painless.

Is a "classical" description of the pain diagnostic?

No. Several other conditions might present in a similar fashion. It would be foolhardy, though, to ignore it!

What additional historical factors might add to the likelihood that this patient is having a myocardial infarction?

A **PAST HISTORY** of

- Angina pectoris
- Previously documented myocardial infarction
- Previously documented hypertension, diabetes, hypercholesterolemia, polycythemia vera, or essential thrombocythemia
- Previous cerebrovascular or occlusive peripheral vascular disease

A **FAMILY HISTORY** of

- Ischemic heart disease
- Cerebrovascular accidents
- Occlusive peripheral vascular disease
- Sudden death
- Diabetes mellitus
- Hypercholesterolemia

A **LIFE SITUATION** involving

- A tense "type A" personality involved in a high-tension occupation
- Recent financial, occupational, or domestic problems

In relation to **CIGARETTE SMOKING**

- A significant smoking history

How may the PHYSICAL EXAMINATION contribute?

An orderly physical examination might reveal

1. From the General Appearance

- An acutely ill patient who is cold, sweating, anxious and restless; who may be belching and vomiting; and who seems pale.

(These features are also compatible with pulmonary embolism, dissection, pancreatitis, or biliary colic, all of which may present with chest pain).

2. With Regard to the Vital Signs

- Tachypnea
- Tachycardia (usually), bradycardia, or an arrhythmia
- Hypotension (or hypertension)

3. In the Head and Neck

- Xanthelasmata of the eyelids
- Fundal changes of diabetes or hypertension
- Characteristic ear lobe creases
- Carotid artery bruits

These features of "risk-factors" increase the likelihood of ischemic disease.

- Moderate elevation of the jugular venous pressure

4. Over the Lung Fields

- Basal crackles

5. In the Precordium

- On inspection and palpation:
  - A prominent and laterally displaced apex beat—evidence of hypertensive cardiomegaly, and, as such, a risk factor
  - Abnormal precordial pulsation, indicating left ventricular segmental dysfunction
- On auscultation:
  - An S3 or S4 gallop rhythm—sometimes detected only with posturing in the left lateral position
  - A paradoxical S2
  - A systolic murmur at the apex or left sternal border

6. In the Extremities

- Evidence of risk factors in the form of
  - Bruits over the femoral arteries
  - Other signs of occlusive peripheral vascular disease
  - Hypercholesterolemic thickening of the tendo-achilles

What laboratory studies are indicated?

- An electrocardiogram

If this is noncontributory, and there is a strong suspicion of an infarction on clinical grounds, the patient should be admitted to a coronary care unit for

- Cardiac monitoring, and
- Specific enzyme studies

What other causes of central chest pain are critical and demand urgent attention?

- Dissecting aneurysm of the aorta
- Pulmonary embolism
- Upper thoracic spinal cord and root compression

What additional factors in the history and physical examination should alert you to the possibility of a DISSECTING ANEURYSM?

With regard to

1. **The Description of the Pain**
   - A "tearing" quality
   - A progressive radiation to the neck, back, abdomen, and lumbar region
   - Prolonged persistence of the pain

2. **The Past History**
   - Prior documentation of Marfan's syndrome, or hypertension —disorders which will predipose to the development of a dissecting aneurysm

3. **The General Appearance**
   - The characteristic tall, thin habitus of Marfan's syndrome

4. **The Mental Status**
   - Loss of consciousness—without evidence of hypotension or an arrhythmia

5. **The Vital Signs**—as assessed from careful examination and *reexamination*:
   - Asymmetric diminution in the intensity of the radial, carotid, and femoral pulses

- Asymmetric diminution of the blood pressure in the arms and legs, especially if such asymmetry should develop over a few hours
- Persistence of severe hypertension
- Pulsus paradoxus, suggesting complicating pericardial hemorrhage and tamponade

6. **The Hands**

- Arachnodactyly—suggesting Marfan's syndrome

7. **The Head**

- Dolichocephaly, a high arched palate, and subluxation of the lens—all suggestive of Marfan's syndrome or one of its variations

8. **The Neck**

- Elevated jugular venous pressure
- Rapid "y" descent
- Kussmaul's sign

—indicating pericardial tamponade complicating pericardial hemorrhage.

9. **The Precordium**

- An early diastolic murmur of aortic incompetence
- A pericardial friction rub

10. **The Thorax**

- Signs of a pleural effusion (hemothorax)

What laboratory studies would increase this suspicion?

- Urinalysis revealing hematuria
- Chest radiographs showing a progressively widening mediastinum, a pleural effusion, or increasing cardiomegaly

What features might suggest PULMONARY EMBOLISM in this man?

With regard to

1. **The PRESENTING ILLNESS**

- A prominent complaint of
  ○ Dyspnea, and/or
  ○ Syncope

2. A SYSTEMS REVIEW relevant to the

- Cardiovascular system
  ○ Pain and/or swelling of a lower limb
- Respiratory system
  ○ Pleuritic chest pain
  ○ Hemoptysis, and/or
  ○ Wheezing

3. The PAST HISTORY or PROBLEM LIST

- Prior documentation of
  ○ Pulmonary embolism, or
  ○ Deep vein thrombosis
- The presence of circumstances or disorders known to predispose to the development of deep vein thrombosis, hence pulmonary embolism, *e.g.*,
  ○ Recent surgery or fracture
  ○ Prolonged bed rest or immobilization
  ○ Prolonged car or airplane travel
  ○ Malignant disease
  ○ Congestive cardiac failure
  ○ Polycythemia vera
  ○ Essential thrombocythemia
- Previous episodes of
  ○ Acute dyspnea, pleuritic chest pain or hemoptysis—suggesting previous embolism

4. The PHYSICAL EXAMINATION, relevant to

- **The vital signs**
  ○ Tachypnea
  ○ Tachycardia
  ○ Hypotension
- **The head and neck**
  ○ Cyanosis
  ○ Elevation of the jugular venous pressure, and the presence of prominent a waves

- **The chest**
  - Localized or generalized wheezing
  - A pleural friction rub
  - Perhaps signs of consolidation
- **The precordium**
  - A palpable lift over the right ventricle
  - A palpable P2
  - A loud P2
  - A Graham Steell murmur of functional pulmonary incompetence
  - A right atrial gallop rhythm at the lower left sternal border, increasing with inspiration
- **The extremities**
  - Signs of a deep vein thrombosis: swelling, warmth, or tenderness of a limb

What additional laboratory studies are indicated?

- A chest radiograph
- A lung scan
- Arterial blood gas determinations

What features should alert you to the possibility of ROOT or CORD COMPRESSION?

1. **A HISTORY of**

- **Pain**
  - Occurring primarily in the back, or seeming to radiate around the chest
  - Exacerbated by movement, coughing, or sneezing

2. **A SYSTEMS REVIEW relevant to the** CENTRAL NERVOUS SYSTEM **which reveals**

- Weakness, paresthesia, and/or numbness in the extremities
- Pain in the extremities with neck flexion
- Loss of bladder and/or bowel control

3. **A PAST HISTORY which includes**

- A diagnosis of malignant disease
- Trauma to the spine

4. **Physical findings of**
   - **In the chest**
     - Tenderness to percussion over the spine
     - An area of hyperesthesia of the chest wall
     - A "sensory level" on the chest wall
   - **In the abdomen**
     - A distended bladder
   - **In the extremities**
     - Signs of cord compression:
       Bilateral upper motor neuron paralysis of the legs: hypotonia (in this early acute phase); paresis or paralysis; hyporeflexia; extensor plantar responses
       Loss of all modalities of sensation in the legs.
   - **On rectal examination**
     - A patulous anus
     - Loss of the anal reflex

What laboratory studies are indicated?

- Radiograph of the thoracic spine
- Perhaps a myelogram

What are the other disorders that can closely mimic the pain of these serious conditions?

These include:

1. **Diseases of the Gastrointestinal Tract**
   - Esophagospasm
   - Esophagitis
   - Hiatus hernia
   - Peptic ulcer
   - Pancreatitis, and
   - Biliary tract disease

2. Disorders of the Chest Wall

- Muscular pain
- Costochondritis
- Disorders of the sternum and ribs

3. Other Disorders of the Heart

- Pericarditis
- Angina pectoris

4. Psychoneurotic Disease

Once the more urgent disorders considered above have been excluded, or while the patient is being observed and investigated for these possibilities, it becomes important that these latter conditions also be considered. As usual, this is best approached first with a careful history and physical examination.

How might the HISTORY help in this regard?

THE DESCRIPTION OF THE PAIN might reveal:

- A more predominantly epigastric *distribution*—a little more suggestive of gastrointestinal tract disease
- *Radiation* to an area beneath the right scapula—suggesting biliary tract disease
- *A colicky quality* to the pain—also suggesting biliary tract disease
- *Precipitation* of the pain by exercise—suggesting angina pectoris; by meals—peptic ulcer disease; by bending forward, or lying flat—hiatus hernia
- *Aggravation* of the pain by movement—suggesting musculoskeletal disease; or by respiration—pericarditis
- *Relief* of the pain by rest, suggesting angina pectoris; by a change in posture—pericardial, pancreatic, or musculoskeletal disease

THE SYSTEMS REVIEW might reveal, with regard to

- **The gastrointestinal tract**
  - ○ Recent dietary indiscretion
  - ○ Excess alcohol consumption

○ Heartburn
○ Dyspeptic symptoms
○ Jaundice
○ Hematemesis or
○ Melena

—all suggesting gastrointestinal tract disease.

THE PAST HISTORY might reveal

● Prior documentation of
○ Biliary tract disease
○ Peptic ulcer disease
○ Hiatus hernia
○ Pancreatitis

which must suggest a possible recurrence.

● Evidence of
○ Trauma to the chest wall or back, suggesting musculo-skeletal disease
○ Previous psychoneurotic disease or personality traits rendering a psychogenic cause for the pain more plausible

A review of **THE LIFE SITUATION** might reveal

● Recent unusual physical exertion that might account for chest wall pain
● Occupational, domestic, financial, or other concerns that might be responsible for psychoneurotic chest pain

How might the PHYSICAL EXAMINATION help?

1. **General Appearance**

    ● If the patient were obese, more especially if the patient were female, this might suggest biliary tract disease.
    ● Jaundice might also suggest biliary tract disease.

2. **Examination of the Chest**

    ● Tenderness over the costochondral junction, ribs, sternum, or muscles, would suggest chest wall disease, as would local swelling or redness.
    ● A pericardial friction rub would indicate pericarditis.

3. Examination of the Abdomen

- Tenderness or guarding would favor intra-abdominal pathology.

What laboratory studies are indicated?

These will depend upon the diagnostic suspicions.

CHAPTER 6

Vomiting

This is a common symptom that may occur in a very large number of disorders—sometimes as the presenting or dominant manifestation of a significant underlying disorder.

It is an unpleasant symptom that often requires symptomatic control, and it may have important consequences.

CAUSES OF VOMITING

How might you reasonably begin to approach the problem of vomiting in a particular patient in order to try to establish its cause?

- By being alert to the more probable causes that are suggested from a review of *that* patient's *problem list.*
- By developing a practical and functional classification of the common and critical causes of vomiting; then directing the orderly history and physical examination toward detecting the "clues" that will enable you to develop an appropriate differential diagnosis for that patient.

How might the review of the PROBLEM LIST contribute to the differential diagnosis of vomiting?

A patient with a previous diagnosis of (for example) *heart failure* would be especially liable to both

- Digitalis toxicity and
- Recurrence of the failure

as causes for vomiting.

A known *diabetic* would be at risk for

- Ketoacidosis

In a patient with *sarcoidosis*

- Hypercalcemia

would need careful consideration.

How might you reasonably and functionally classify the more common, and the critical, causes of nausea and vomiting?

It is useful in this regard to consider these symptoms as arising from

1. Disorders of the Gastrointestinal Tract

- Inflammatory lesions of the
  - Stomach
  - Duodenum
  - Gall bladder
  - Liver
  - Pancreas
  - Appendix or
  - Small or large bowel
- Obstructive lesions of the
  - Stomach or duodenum
  - Small bowel or
  - Large bowel

2. Disorders of the Genitourinary Tract

- Inflammatory disease of the urinary tract or pelvic organs
- Obstructive disorders of the urinary tract, *e.g.*, ureteric stone
- Testicular torsion or trauma
- Pregnancy
- Dysmenorrhea

3. Disorders of the Central Nervous System

- Psychogenic factors
- Migraine
- Cerebrovascular disease

- Meningitis and encephalitis
- Inner ear disease
- Space-occupying intracranial lesions

4. **Metabolic Abnormalities.** The underlying causes might include:

  - Exogenous toxins
    - Chemical agents, such as *drugs* or *poisons*
    - Physical agents, such as *radiotherapy* or *sunburn*
  - Endogenous toxins, from *renal failure, liver failure,* or *acute porphyria*
  - Endocrine disorders, such as *diabetic ketoacidosis* or *hypoadrenalism*
  - Electrolyte imbalance: *hyponatremia* or *hypercalcemia*

5. **Infection**

  - Localized or
  - Systemic

6. **Other "Reflex" Causes**

  - With myocardial infarction
  - With severe pain
  - Following extreme physical exertion
  - In congestive cardiac failure

Utilizing this classification, what symptoms would it be reasonable to consider in trying to develop a differential diagnosis for a patient who is vomiting?

An analysis of the **CHARACTERISTICS** of the vomiting might be contributory. With regard to

1. **Its Onset, Course, and Duration**

  - A long history of frequent vomiting, easily provoked, in an otherwise healthy patient would suggest a psychogenic basis.
  - Morning nausea and vomiting, occurring on a daily basis in a young woman, would be very suggestive of pregnancy or oral contraceptive use. It would also suggest alcoholic gastritis (in either sex).

- Repeated "attacks" of nausea and vomiting—associated with *abdominal pain*—would suggest
  - Biliary tract disease
  - Pancreatitis, and perhaps
  - Appendicitis
  - Intermittent intestinal obstruction
  - Ureteric obstruction, or
  - Dysmenorrhea
- Other conditions that might be associated with recurrent episodes of nausea and vomiting include
  - Migraine
  - Meniere's disease
  - Transient ischemic attacks
- An acute onset of significant nausea and vomiting would suggest
  - Gastritis, with an infectious, toxic, or allergic cause
- If such nausea and vomiting were associated with abdominal pain,
  - Acute appendicitis
  - Acute cholecystitis
  - Acute pancreatitis
  - Intestinal obstruction, and perhaps
  - Diabetic ketoacidosis, and
  - Acute intermittent porphyria

—would all need particular consideration.

- The following conditions might also need to be considered in the patient with an acute onset of vomiting:
  - Meningitis
  - Encephalitis
  - Migraine
  - Labyrinthitis
  - A cerebrovascular accident
  - Acute myocardial infarction, and
  - An infection—especially in a child
- The development of persistent and perhaps increasing nausea and vomiting over several weeks would suggest
  - Peptic ulcer disease
  - Gastric carcinoma

○ Large bowel obstruction
○ A space-occupying intracranial lesion
○ Metabolic disorders—especially *drugs, poisons, renal failure, liver failure, hypercalcemia*

2. Its Quantity and Quality

• Vast amounts of vomitus, or the presence of undigested food from a previous meal in the vomitus, would suggest a pyloric obstruction.
• Residues of drugs in the vomitus would suggest acute poisoning and drug overdosage.
• Feculent vomitus would suggest a late diagnosis of intestinal obstruction.
• Visible blood, or a "coffee grounds" appearance to the vomitus—hematemesis—has very special implications. The approach to such a patient would be quite different and is not considered further in this chapter.

Further enquiry into the **HISTORY,** with careful consideration of its several components, will usually reveal information of diagnostic significance, as shown in Table 6-1.

On the basis of the "diagnostic clues" elicited from the **HISTORY,** a differential diagnosis will usually become apparent.

The **HISTORY, PHYSICAL EXAMINATION,** and laboratory studies can then be directed toward establishing a firm diagnosis, as illustrated in the following case studies.

CASE STUDIES

A 16-year-old girl is brought to her family doctor by her mother because she has felt nauseated and has vomited after breakfast each morning for the past 2 weeks. She is otherwise well.

What are the probable causes?

• Pregnancy is very likely.
• Oral contraception is possible.

TABLE 6-1. SYMPTOMS OF POTENTIAL DIAGNOSTIC SIGNIFICANCE IN A PATIENT WHO IS VOMITING

Source	Symptom	Potential diagnostic significance
Review of systems		
GASTROINTESTINAL SYSTEM	Dietary intake Excessive quantity Excessive alcohol Unusual foodstuffs Possible contamination of food	Gastric irritation or Gastritis
	An absence of nausea	CNS disease
	Dyspeptic symptoms	Peptic ulcer disease A gastric carcinoma Cholelithiasis and cholecystitis

	Abdominal pain	Disorders of the gastrointestinal tract—
		    irritative
		    inflammatory or
		    obstructive
		Renal colic
		Pyelonephritis and salpingitis
		Dysmenorrhea
		Testicular torsion or trauma
		Diabetic ketoacidosis

	Jaundice	Hepatitis Biliary tract disease Hepatic metastases
	Diarrhea	Gastroenteritis Acute appendicitis Pyelonephritis Salpingitis
	Constipation	Intestinal obstruction Ileus due to inflammatory disease
THE GENITO-URINARY SYSTEM	Frequency of urination	Early pregnancy
	Dysuria and frequency	A urinary tract infection Acute appendicitis Other intra-abdominal pelvic or inflammatory disease
	Polyuria	Hypercalcemia Chronic renal failure Diabetic ketoacidosis
	Hematuria	Urinary tract disease
THE CENTRAL NERVOUS SYSTEM	Headache	Migraine
	Convulsions	A systemic infection
	Loss of consciousness	Meningoencephalitis
	Visual disturbances	A cerebrovascular accident
	Localizing CNS symptoms	A space-occupying intracranial lesion
	Tinnitus or Vertigo	Acute labyrinthitis Meniere's disease A cerebrovascular accident

(continued)

TABLE 6-1. SYMPTOMS OF POTENTIAL DIAGNOSTIC SIGNIFICANCE IN A PATIENT WHO IS VOMITING (*Continued*)

Source	Symptom	Potential diagnostic significance
THE CARDIO-VASCULAR SYSTEM	Chest pain Dyspnea Palpitations Syncope	Myocardial infarction
GENERAL HEALTH	Fever	An infection A cerebrovascular accident
The past history	Previous abdominal surgery Recent head trauma Previous gastrointestinal, genitourinary, CNS, or metabolic disease	Intestinal bands, or adhesions causing obstruction A subdural hematoma Recurrence or progression of the disease
The family history	Concurrent nausea and vomiting in other family members	Toxic or infective gastroenteritis
The life situation	Personal, family, or occupational problems Occupational or other exposure to toxins or infectious agents	Psychogenic vomiting
Medications	Careful documentation of *all* medications and treatment, including radiation therapy, is indicated.	Gastric irritation Central effects
Alcohol consumption and drug addiction	Alcohol consumption —acute or chronic excess	Acute gastritis Acute pancreatitis Chronic relapsing pancreatitis Acute alcoholic hepatitis A subdural hematoma—because of the greater liability of the alcoholic to trauma Infection—greater liability in the alcoholic A brain tumor—causing both the vomiting and the alcoholism
	Drug use	Drug toxicity Withdrawal effects Viral hepatitis Infection

How would you confirm the cause?

This will require a very tactful **HISTORY**. There may be, with regard to

- The **genitourinary system**
  - Amenorrhea and
  - Frequency of micturition
- The **breasts**
  - Fullness and tingling of the nipples
- The **life situation**
  - Appropriate exposure
- **Medications**
  - Oral contraceptive usage

A *vaginal* **EXAMINATION** might well yield additional useful information, but is probably not indicated.

Laboratory tests can confirm pregnancy. If *negative*, they should be repeated after 1-2 weeks.

A 24-year-old male student is brought into the emergency room because of severe nausea and vomiting that has begun 3-4 hours previously. Further questioning reveals that he has had abdominal pain over this same period. He had consumed a large meal and a "moderate" amount of alcohol prior to the onset of these symptoms. He had previously been in good health. His father is a diabetic. None of his colleagues is similarly afflicted.

What is a reasonable differential diagnosis in this patient?

- Acute gastritis. This is by far the most likely cause in a young adult who has overindulged. Food poisoning is unlikely, since nobody else has similar symptoms.

There are a number of other conditions that *must* be carefully considered because of their therapeutic implications:

- Acute appendicitis. This is suggested by the association of nausea, vomiting, and abdominal pain.
- Acute pancreatitis. This condition is further suggested by the food and alcohol excesses.
- Diabetic ketoacidosis. The possibility of this condition must be considered in view of the family history of diabetes.

How might you differentiate among these disorders—from the HISTORY?

A more detailed description of the pain may reveal the characteristic features of

1. Acute Appendicitis

- *Site:* Initially periumbilical
- *Radiation:* Later localizing in the right iliac fossa
- *Character:* Initially colicky; later continuous
- *Severity:* Mild to moderate
- *Aggravating features:* Worse with jolting or movement

2. Acute Pancreatitis

- *Site:* Epigastric; right or left upper quadrants or whole upper abdomen
- *Radiation:* Through to the back, or left side
- *Severity:* Moderate to marked
- *Relieving features:* Characteristic flexed posture

3. Diabetic Ketoacidosis

- *Site:* Diffuse
- *Severity:* Marked

4. Acute Gastritis

- *Site:* Epigastric

How might you differentiate among these disorders—from the PHYSICAL EXAMINATION?

Features suggesting one or another of these disorders may be present. The potential findings in each should be considered, in an orderly, routine fashion, as listed below:

1. Acute Appendicitis

- General Appearance
  - ○ Gait: a slightly stooped posture when walking
  - ○ Posture: slight flexion of the right hip
- Vital Signs: pyrexia, tachycardia
- Head and Neck: flushing of the cheeks
- The Abdomen

- On inspection: diminished abdominal-wall movement
- On palpation: tenderness, guarding, and rigidity—in the right iliac fossa
- On percussion: tenderness to light percussion (a more gentle technique for eliciting the rebound tenderness of peritonitis) over the right iliac fossa

In the absence of anterior abdominal signs, the following findings might be evident:

- On rectal examination
  - Localized tenderness to palpation, if the appendix lay over the brim of the pelvis
- On examination of the extremities
  - Pain on hyperextension of the hip, if the appendix were retrocecal

2. Acute Pancreatitis

- General Appearance
  - A distressed patient who looks very ill
- Vital Signs
  - Fever
  - Hypotension
- The Abdomen
  - On palpation: Tenderness and guarding, but with much less rigidity than might have been anticipated from the severity of the pain.

3. Diabetic Ketoacidosis

- Mental Status
  - Drowsiness and confusion
- Vital Signs
  - Hypotension
  - Kussmaul's respirations
  - Tachycardia
- The Head
  - The eyes: Flaccidity of the eyeballs
  - The breath: A ketotic odor
  - The mouth: Dryness of the tongue and mucous membranes

- The Skin
  - Loss of tissue turgor

4. **Acute Gastritis.** There may be evidence of some epigastric tenderness, but otherwise very little that is abnormal will be detected.

What laboratory tests would be appropriate?

- A complete blood count, especially the total and differential leukocyte cell counts
- Urinalysis—seeking evidence of glycosuria and ketonuria
- Assays for serum concentration of amylase and glucose, and a test for ketonemia
- Urinary amylase quantitation
- Abdominal radiographs

One of your assignments in the Physical Diagnosis Course is to interview a 43-year-old female patient who has recently been admitted to the hospital for investigation of increasing bone pain.

During the "systems review" she mentions that she has been nauseated over the past 7–8 days and that she has vomited several times during this period.

Upon further questioning, you learn that the patient was diagnosed as having a carcinoma of the left breast 6 years previously, and that this was treated by mastectomy followed by local radiotherapy. Three years later she was found to have bony metastases, and was treated successfully with oophorectomy.

She is now in reasonably good health, apart from the bone pain and the nausea and vomiting that she mentioned to you.

Do the nausea and vomiting warrant elevation to problem status, and hence further consideration in this patient?

Despite the fact that they were not of sufficient significance to the patient to complain about them directly, their diagnostic implications in a patient with known malignant disease are such that they must be pursued.

What causes for vomiting need particular consideration in this patient?

A patient with **KNOWN BREAST CANCER** would be especially likely to vomit because of

1. **Metastatic disease, with involvement of**

   - The *gastrointestinal tract,* producing intestinal obstruction
   - The *liver,* causing liver failure
   - The *brain or meninges,* causing increased intracranial pressure
   - The *ureters,* causing obstructive renal failure

2. **The side effects of treatment**

   - Radiotherapy
   - Hormonal therapy
   - Chemotherapy, and/or
   - Analgesics

   Any of these could be responsible for vomiting.

3. **Other consequences of the disease and its treatment, especially**

   - Hypercalcemia and
   - Opportunistic infection

How might the HISTORY contribute to establishing the specific diagnosis?

1. **Intestinal obstruction might be suggested by evidence of:**

   - In the Gastrointestinal System
     - Colicky abdominal pain
     - Abdominal distention, and/or
     - Constipation

2. **Hepatic metastases by complaints of:**

   - Jaundice, and/or
   - Right upper quadrant discomfort

3. **Intracranial metastases by symptoms relevant to:**

   - The Central Nervous System
     - Headache
     - Convulsions

- ○ Altered consciousness
- ○ Visual disturbances
- ○ Disturbances of speech or swallowing
- ○ Disturbances of balance or coordination
- ○ Parasthesias, or
- ○ Weakness of a limb

The presence of such symptoms in a patient with advanced breast cancer might also indicate meningeal infection—often by opportunistic agents such as *Candida, Cryptococcus,* or *Listeria.*

The potential role of the patient's **therapy** can be explored by a careful review of the details relevant to *her drug therapy and management.*

How might the orderly PHYSICAL EXAMINATION contribute to establishing the diagnosis?

With regard to

1. The Vital Signs

- • Hypodrenalism would be suggested by hypotension.

2. The Hand

- • Significant liver involvement, and perhaps renal failure, might be reflected by a flapping tremor.

3. The Mental Status

- • An abnormal mental status would be a useful clue to
  - ○ Brain metastases
  - ○ Meningeal involvement by tumor or infection
  - ○ Renal or hepatic failure
  - ○ Hypercalcemia

4. The Head. Examination is useful for the diagnosis of

- • Cerebral metastases
- • Meningeal involvement by tumor, or opportunistic infection —from evidence of
  - ○ Papilloedema, and perhaps
  - ○ Cranial nerve palsies
- • Liver failure—from the presence of

○ Fetor hepaticus, and

○ Jaundice

5. **The Neck.** Examination of the neck might further support a diagnosis of *meningeal involvement* by tumor or infection, as indicated by

- Neck stiffness, and
- Brudzinski's sign

6. **The Abdomen.** Examination of the abdomen is important to the diagnosis of

- *Metastatic liver disease,* where the following conditions may be found:
  ○ Hepatomegaly
  ○ A hepatic friction rub, and/or
  ○ A bruit over the liver
- *Intestinal obstruction,* where the following signs might be apparent:
  ○ A distended abdomen
  ○ Visible peristalsis
  ○ A tympanitic percussion note
  ○ Increased bowel sounds

7. **The Extremities.** Central nervous system metastases or infection might be suggested by

- Involuntary movements
- Increased muscle tone
- Weakness
- Incoordination
- Sensory abnormalities
- Altered reflexes in the limbs

What laboratory studies are indicated in this patient in order to help establish the diagnosis?

Serum concentrations of

- BUN, creatinine
- Bilirubin, alkaline phosphatase, SGOT
- Calcium
- Sodium and potassium

should always be determined.

Judicious studies to confirm the clinical impression already gained might include

- Abdominal radiographs
- Computerized axial tomography of the brain
- A lumbar puncture (be careful!)
- Adrenal steroid studies

EFFECTS OF VOMITING

What are the potential consequences of prolonged, or severe, vomiting?

- Fluid and electrolyte loss
- Alkalosis
- Aspiration of vomitus
- An esophageal tear

How may these consequences of vomiting be detected from the history and physical examination?

The following features would suggest:

1. Aspiration

- Complaints of cough and dyspnea
- The presence of a fever
- Signs of pulmonary consolidation

2. Fluid and Electrolyte Loss

- Symptoms and signs of dehydration
  - A diminished urinary output
  - Hypotension and tachycardia
  - Loss of skin turgor
  - Flaccidity of the eyeballs
  - Dryness of the mouth and tongue

3. Alkalosis

- Positive Chvostek and Trousseau signs
- Carpopedal spasm

- An abnormal mental status
  - Apathy
  - Confusion
  - Stupor

4. An Esophageal Tear

- A history of hematemesis occurring after prolonged or strenuous vomiting

CHAPTER 7

Polyuria

A 28-year-old patient complains to you that for the past month she has been both drinking and passing excessive amounts of fluid.

Is this likely to be clinically meaningful?

Yes, particularly since these are symptoms of recent onset, persistent over a month, and sufficiently bothersome for her to consult a physician. Her description suggests polydipsia and polyuria—symptoms that are often significant.

What is polyuria?

Polyuria refers to the voiding of an excessive volume of urine—usually more than 2.5–3.0 litres a day.

How does polyuria manifest?

- With an increase in both the *volume* and *frequency* of micturition. (Polyuria is one of several causes of "frequency")
- With *nocturia*—since frequency is usually more apparent at night
- With *thirst* and *polydipsia*—as a consequence of the polyuria

How may polyuria be confirmed?

- By a careful history, in which an attempt is made to quantitate the frequency and volume of urination and of fluid intake
- By collecting and measuring the 24-hour urine output

What is its significance?

- Polyuria may result in dehydration.
- It may constitute a clue to significant underlying pathology.

CAUSES OF POLYURIA

What circumstances might account for polyuria?

- It could constitute a physiologic response to a variety of factors.
- It is to be anticipated in a number of clinical situations.
- It may be the presenting symptom in several specific disease states.

Under what "physiologic" circumstances might polyuria occur?

- During cold weather
- With anxiety
- With increased fluid intake—especially beer, other forms of alcohol, tea, or coffee. This will be particularly noticeable if such intake occurs just before bedtime.

Under what clinical circumstances might urine output be expected to increase?

- In the "unloading" of edema fluid, as in
  - The treatment of congestive cardiac failure with bed rest alone, and/or with diuretics
  - Cyclic edema related to the menstrual cycle, which may be associated with noticeable cyclic polyuria
- Following treatment with diuretics. This would apply even in the nonedematous patient, such as a hypertensive subject on diuretics for the control of hypertension.
- In the recovery phase of acute tubular necrosis; or
- Following the relief of an obstructive uropathy

What significant clinical disorders might present with, or manifest, polyuria?

- Diabetes mellitus

- Diabetes insipidus
- Chronic renal failure
- Hypercalcemia
- Hypokalemia
- Psychogenic polydipsia

Your patient describes getting out of bed three or four times each night to urinate. The volume seems considerable, since the flow persists for 20-30 seconds. She would previously urinate at most once during the night.

Over the same period she has been drinking five or six glasses of water during the day—something quite unusual for her.

In all probability, therefore, she does indeed have polyuria and polydipsia.

Utilizing a knowledge of the likely causes, how might you try to establish the diagnosis?

A review of the **PROBLEM LIST** might reveal prior documentation of disorders that would *increase the likelihood* that one or another of the disease states under consideration is present. For example:

- A villous adenoma of the bowel is likely to be associated with hypokalemia, as is chronic diarrhea, or primary aldosteronism.
- Malignant disease might be complicated by hypercalcemia, or metastatic involvement of the posterior pituitary gland.
- Sarcoidosis might similarly be complicated by hypercalcemia or posterior pituitary disease.
- Head trauma, meningitis, or other intracranial disease is likely to be associated with diabetes insipidus.

The **STRUCTURED INTERVIEW** might be geared toward seeking those symptoms or clues that indicate or suggest one or another of these various disorders, as detailed in Table 7-1.

On interviewing the patient further you learn that she has felt increasingly tired over the past month, and that she has lost about 5 lbs in weight during this time. (She is not trying to diet).

Her prescription lenses have needed changing twice in the past 4 months.

Her father died at the age of 48 of a myocardial infarction. She has one child, age 8, who weighed 10 lbs 4 oz at birth. She has had two miscarriages.

TABLE 7-1. INFORMATION OF POTENTIAL SIGNIFICANCE IN A PATIENT WITH POLYURIA

Source	Symptom	Potential significance
Review of systems		
GENERAL HEALTH	Weight loss	Diabetes mellitus
	Lassitude and fatigue	Diabetes mellitus
		Chronic renal disease
		Diabetes insipidus
		Psychogenic polydipsia
	Profound weakness	Hypokalemia
GASTROIN-TESTINAL SYSTEM	Anorexia	Hypercalcemia
	Nausea	Chronic renal disease
	Vomiting	
	Polyphagia	Diabetes mellitus
	Preference for ice-cold water	Diabetes insipidus
	Hiccoughs	Chronic renal disease
	Ingestion of large volumes of tea, coffee, alcohol	Probable basis for "physiologic" polyuria
	Constipation	Hypercalcemia
		Hypokalemia
THE SKIN	Recurrent carbuncles and furuncles	Diabetes mellitus
	Pruritus	Chronic renal disease
		Diabetes mellitus
	Easy bruising	Chronic renal disease
GENITOURI-NARY SYSTEM	Infertility	Diabetes mellitus
	Pruritus vulvae	Diabetes mellitus
	Impotence (in a man) and loss of libido	Diabetes mellitus
		Perhaps a clue to psychogenic polydipsia
	Dysuria	Diabetes mellitus (urinary tract infection)
NERVOUS SYSTEM	Drowsiness	Hypercalcemia
		Chronic renal disease
		Diabetes mellitus
	Blurring of vision	Diabetes mellitus
	Diplopia	
	Headache	Diabetes insipidus
	Visual field defect	
PSYCHO-LOGICAL STATUS	Anxiety	Anxiety-induced polydipsia
Past history		
PREVIOUS ILLNESSES	Prior documentation of: Renal disease Diabetes mellitus Diabetes insipidus Hypercalcemia Hypokalemia Psychogenic polydipsia	Obvious!? But how humiliating to discover that you have overlooked such obvious factors after days or weeks of searching.

(continued)

TABLE 7-1. INFORMATION OF POTENTIAL SIGNIFICANCE IN A PATIENT WITH POLYURIA (*Continued*)

Source	Symptom	Potential significance
	Meningitis Encephalitis Cerebrovascular accident	Diabetes insipidus
PSYCHIATRIC ILLNESSES	Depression Psychoneurotic illness Anorexia nervosa Personality disorder	Psychogenic polydipsia Anxiety-induced polyuria
OBSTETRICAL EVENTS	Infertility Repeated miscarriages Toxemia of pregnancy Hydramnios Stillbirths Large babies, with birth weights in excess of 10 lbs Respiratory distress syndrome in neonates	Diabetes mellitus
TRAUMA	Head injury	Diabetes insipidus
Family history		
	Diabetes mellitus, or complications of diabetes mellitus, *e.g.*, atherosclerotic vascular disease in close family members	Diabetes mellitus
Current life situation		
	Poor job record Poor marriage record Social problems Conflict with the law	Psychogenic polydipsia Alcohol-induced polyuria Anxiety
Medication and treatment history		
	Use of diuretics Analgesic abuse Antacid excesses Steroid administration Lithium carbonate or demeclocycline use Brain surgery or radiation therapy	Diuresis and resultant polyuria Hypokalemia Chronic renal disease Hypercalcemia Hypokalemia Diabetes insipidus (nephrogenic) Diabetes insipidus
Alcohol use		
	Alcohol at bedtime Excess alcohol consumption	Alcohol-induced polyuria

What is the probable diagnosis?

Diabetes mellitus must be suggested by the constellation of weight loss, visual problems, abnormal obstetric history, and family history of atherosclerotic disease.

PHYSICAL FINDINGS IN DIABETES MELLITUS

What signs in the orderly PHYSICAL EXAMINATION would you specifically seek in further support of this diagnosis?

With regard to

1. Her General Appearance

   - Obesity, *or*
   - Evidence of weight loss

2. The Skin

   - Carotinodermia
   - Furuncles and carbuncles

3. The Eyes

   - Xanthelasmata of the eyelids
   - A diabetic retinopathy, involving, even at this early stage, any or all of the following:
     - Microaneurysms
     - Hemorrhages
     - Small, hard exudates
     - "Cotton wool" spots

4. The Genitalia

   - A monilial vaginitis

5. The Extremities

   - Necrobiosis lipoidica diabeticorum
   - Absent ankle jerks (an early sign of a polyneuropathy)

What confirmatory laboratory studies are indicated?

- Urinalysis—looking for *glycosuria*

- Fasting and 2-hour postprandial blood glucose assays—looking for hyperglycemia

If diabetes mellitus were not confirmed, what would you do?

- The diagnosis is so likely that the tests should be repeated.
- It would, however, also be appropriate to examine the patient again, looking for evidence of the other disorders that are being considered, and to arrange appropriate laboratory studies.

What signs would you now look for in the orderly PHYSICAL EXAMINATION?

With regard to

1. **Her General Appearance**
   - Weight loss, which might indicate chronic renal disease, as might the detection of an ammoniacal odour.

2. **Her Mental Status**
   - Drowsiness and/or irritability, which would suggest chronic renal disease or hypercalcemia (or ketosis).

3. **Her Vital Signs**
   - Hypertension, which would suggest
     - Chronic renal disease
     - Primary aldosteronism, or
     - Cushing's syndrome
   - Kussmaul's (acidotic), respirations, which would strongly suggest chronic renal failure (provided she is *not* ketotic).

4. **Her Skin**
   - A sallow complexion and/or bruising, which would suggest chronic renal disease

5. **Her Head**
   - Bitemporal hemianopia, which would suggest diabetes insipidus
   - "Uremic frost," often best seen on the forehead, which would obviously suggest chronic renal disease.

- Pallor of the mucous membranes, which would suggest anemia—as a possible manifestation of chronic renal disease
- Fundal hemorrhages, and evidence of a hypertensive retinopathy, which would also suggest chronic renal disease

6. Her Precordium

- A pericardial friction rub, or
- Evidence of hypertensive heart disease,

which would suggest chronic renal disease.

7. Her Extremities

- Gross tremors, twitching, asterixis, and signs of a peripheral neuropathy, which again would suggest chronic renal disease

What laboratory studies would you arrange?

- Urinalysis—looking for proteinuria and an abnormal urinary sediment
- Serum assays for concentrations of
  - Creatinine and BUN
  - Sodium, potassium, chloride, and bicarbonate
  - Calcium
- Serum and urine osmolality determinations

DEHYDRATION

Irrespective of the *cause* of this patient's polyuria and polydipsia, the potential for her becoming dehydrated, as a *consequence,* is very real.

How may the presence, and even degree, of dehydration be assessed—from the PHYSICAL EXAMINATION?

There may be, with regard to

1. Her Vital Signs

- Hypotension
- Tachycardia

2. Her Head

- Flaccidity of the eyeballs
- Dryness of the tongue and oral mucous membranes

3. Her Skin

- Dryness of the skin, and loss of skin turgor

What laboratory data may be of value in assessing the presence and extent of dehydration?

- Hemoglobin concentration and hematocrit
- Total serum protein concentration
- Serum BUN and creatinine concentrations
- Serum and urine osmolality determinations
- Urine specific gravity
- Urine electrolyte concentrations

DIABETES MELLITUS

Upon further evaluation, you note that the patient does, in fact have glycosuria, and that her fasting blood glucose concentration is 250 mg/dl.

Thus, a diagnosis of diabetes mellitus is confirmed, and the diagnostic process will have progressed from

Polyuria

$\longrightarrow$ *Diabetes mellitus*

The causes and effects of polyuria in the patient have been considered and resolved. However, by achieving a "higher level of resolution" of the problem, it *now* becomes necessary to determine the cause and effects of diabetes mellitus in this patient.

CAUSES

What are the causes of diabetes mellitus?

- Genetic
- Idiopathic
- Drug-induced

- ○ Thiazide diuretics
- ○ Corticosteroids
- ○ L-asparaginase
- • Pancreatic
- ○ Chronic pancreatitis
- ○ Pancreatectomy
- ○ Pancreatic cancer
- ○ Hemochromatosis
- • Endocrine
- ○ Cushing's syndrome
- ○ Acromegaly
- ○ Thyrotoxicosis
- ○ Pheochromocytoma

How might you differentiate among these causes?

A positive **FAMILY HISTORY** for diabetes mellitus would virtually confirm a *genetic* basis.

A **MEDICATION HISTORY** would quickly point to a possible *drug-related* cause.

With regard to possible *pancreatic disease,* a

- • **SYSTEMS REVIEW** relevant to the *gastrointestinal tract* might reveal a history of
  - ○ Abdominal pain—suggestive of pancreatitis, or
  - ○ Abnormal bowel movements—suggestive of malabsorption, hence pancreatitis
- • Review of the **PAST HISTORY** or **PROBLEM LIST** might reveal evidence of
  - ○ Recurrent attacks of abdominal pain, perhaps due to pancreatitis, or
  - ○ A pancreatectomy
- • The **ALCOHOL and DRUG HISTORY** might reveal
  - ○ Excessive alcohol intake, suggesting pancreatitis

With regard to *other pancreatic disorders*

- • *Pancreatic cancer* is very unlikely to present with diabetes-related polyuria; in addition, weight loss, jaundice, and abdominal pain would usually be obvious by this stage.
- • *Hemochromatosis* is often "missed" and is worthy of specific

consideration, even though it would be very unusual in a female. In addition to the symptoms of diabetes mellitus, the **REVIEW OF SYSTEMS** might reveal in

○ The **skin:** a color change
○ The **cardiovascular system:** dyspnea on effort, palpitations, or ankle edema

The **FAMILY HISTORY** might be positive.

PHYSICAL SIGNS might include:

• Increased skin pigmentation
• Hepatomegaly and the signs of chronic liver disease (see Chap. 16)
• The features of heart failure (see Chap. 18)

With regard to the *endocrine disorders:*

• It is only in Cushing's syndrome that the features of diabetes mellitus are likely to be predominant, with polyuria a prominent symptom.

The **PHYSICAL EXAMINATION** might reveal in

• The **general appearance**
  ○ The typical body habitus
• The **mental status**
  ○ Irritability
  ○ Emotional lability
  ○ Depression
  ○ Confusion
  ○ Frank psychosis
• The **vital signs**
  ○ Hypertension
• The **skin**
  ○ Bruising
  ○ Cutaneous striae
• The **head and neck**
  ○ A "moon" facies
  ○ Plethora
  ○ Acne
  ○ Hirsutism
  ○ A "buffalo" hump, or
  ○ Supraclavicular fat pads

Appropriate laboratory tests may be utilized to confirm a clinical suspicion.

EFFECTS

What are the potential effects of diabetes mellitus?

- Diabetic coma
- Ocular complications
- Neuropathic complications
- Vascular disease
- Renal complications
- Skin complications
- Complications of treatment

How may these be detected?

By utilizing an orderly **HISTORY AND PHYSICAL EXAMINATION**, with some appropriate laboratory assistance—as detailed in Table 7-2.

TABLE 7-2. HISTORY AND PHYSICAL EXAMINATION APPROPRIATE TO THE INITIAL AND FOLLOW-UP EVALUATION OF A PATIENT WITH DIABETES MELLITUS

Source	Symptom or sign	Potential significance
Review of systems		
GENERAL HEALTH	Weight loss	Poor diabetic control
	Fatigue, lassitude	
	Fever	Superimposed infection
	Sweating	Hypoglycemia
EENT	Blurring of vision	Cataracts
		Poor control
	Pain in the eye	Oculomotor palsy
		Rubeosis iridis
		Glaucoma
	Diplopia	Oculomotor palsy
CENTRAL NERVOUS SYSTEM	Headache	Hypoglycemia
		Oculomotor palsy
	Drowsiness	
	Irritability	Ketosis
	Faintness	Hyperglycemia
	Loss of consciousness	Hypoglycemia
	Syncope	Postural hypotension (autonomic neuropathy)
	Paresthesia	Peripheral neuropathy
	Numbness	Mononeuritis

(text continues on p. 88)

TABLE 7-2. HISTORY AND PHYSICAL EXAMINATION APPRO-PRIATE TO THE INITIAL AND FOLLOW-UP EVALUATION OF A PATIENT WITH DIABETES MELLITUS (Continued)

Source	Symptom or sign	Potential significance
	Limb pain	Diabetic amyotrophy Peripheral vascular disease
CARDIO- VASCULAR SYSTEM	Chest pain Claudication Edema	Ischemic heart disease Peripheral vascular disease Nephrotic syndrome Hypertension or Ischemic heart failure
GASTROIN- TESTINAL SYSTEM	Nausea Vomiting Abdominal pain Nocturnal diarrhea	Ketosis Autonomic neuropathy
GENITOURI- NARY SYSTEM	Frequency Dysuria Impotence Incontinence	Urinary tract infection Automatic neuropathy
SKIN	Pruritus Rash Skin lesions	Effects of diabetes or insulin therapy
Past history	Myocardial infarction Coma Gangrene and amputation Eye problems Renal disease	
Physical examination		
MENTAL STATUS	Drowsiness Stupor Coma	Ketosis Hyperglycemia coma Hypoglycemia coma
VITAL SIGNS	Hypertension Hypotension Kussmaul's breathing Ketotic odor Pyrexia	Renal disease Dehydration Infection Myocardial infarction Ketosis Infection Dehydration Hypoglycemia
HAND	Dupuytren's contractures	

HEAD
  Eye
	Xanthelasmata
	3rd & 6th nerve palsies
	Rubeosis iridis
	Cataracts
	Retinopathy
	  diabetic
		Cutaneous
		Neurologic
		
		Ocular and
		Vascular complications of diabetes

(continued)

TABLE 7-2. HISTORY AND PHYSICAL EXAMINATION APPRO-
PRIATE TO THE INITIAL AND FOLLOW-UP EVALUATION OF A
PATIENT WITH DIABETES MELLITUS *(Continued)*

Source	Symptom or sign	Potential significance
	proliferative hypertensive	
Mouth	Dehydration	Hyperglycemia
GENITALIA	Vaginitis (or balanitis)	
EXTREMITIES		
Skin	Rubeosis of the feet	Cutaneous effects
	Necrobiosis lipoidica diabeticorum	
Joints	Charcot's joints	Neuropathy
Vascular system	Trophic changes including:	
	ulceration and gangrene	Ischemic disease
	If pulses palpable	Microvascular disease
	Edema	Nephrotic syndrome
		Heart failure
Nervous system	Muscle wasting	Amyotrophy
		Mononeuritis
	Proximal weakness	Proximal myopathy
	Peripheral weakness	
	Peripheral sensory loss	
	Loss of deep tendon reflexes	Peripheral neuropathy
Laboratory investigations		
URINALYSIS	Proteinuria	Renal complications
		Urinary tract infection
	Glycosuria	Reflects quality of control
	Ketonuria	Ketosis
URINE CULTURE	Bacteriuria	Infection
BLOOD GLUCOSE	Hyper- or hypo-glycemia	
SERUM CREATININE, BUN CON-CENTRATIONS	Elevation	Renal failure
		Dehydration

CHAPTER 8

Joint Pain

The diagnostic approach to the patient with joint pain will vary according to several circumstances, since the *probable* causes will also differ.

Thus, in a patient complaining of joint pain it is useful, at the outset, to determine whether

- There is involvement of a single joint, or of multiple joints
- Large joints are affected, or small joints
- The onset is acute, or the process is chronic, recurrent, or progressive
- Symptoms are confined to the joint(s), or systemic symptoms are also present

A 45-year-old female patient is referred to the rheumatology clinic because of "joint pain." As the intern in the clinic, you see her first, and learn that over the past 3 weeks she has noticed increasing discomfort in the middle and ring fingers of both hands. Movement of these fingers is quite painful, and grasping objects is, as a consequence, difficult.

What clinical circumstances could account for these symptoms?

- Disease of the joints—polyarthritis
- Bone disease
- Nerve pathology
- Soft-tissue disease
- Psychogenic disease

POLYARTHRITIS

What clinical findings will allow you to make a diagnosis of polyarthritis?

INSPECTION of the outstretched hand may reveal evidence of

- Swelling of the involved joints

PALPATION may reveal

- Tenderness to pressure over the involved joints, exacerbated or precipitated by simultaneous passive movement of the joint

THE RANGE OF MOVEMENT, both active and passive, may be limited, although sometimes only at the extremes of movement.

If polyarthritis is confirmed as the cause for the pain in her hands, what is a reasonable "next step" in differential diagnosis?

First, differential diagnosis rests between

- A degenerative arthritis—osteoarthritis—and
- The inflammatory polyarthritides

It is useful to confirm or exclude a degenerative process before proceeding further.

OSTEOARTHRITIS

How might a diagnosis of osteoarthritis be confirmed?

The **HISTORY** might be useful, and *should* reveal, with regard to

- Her general health
  - ○ An *absence* of systemic symptoms such as fever, fatigue, lassitude, and weight loss

It *may* reveal, in

- The locomotor system
  - ○ Pain in the distal interphalangeal (DIP) or proximal interphalangeal (PIP) joints, carpometacarpal joints of the

thumbs, or in the hips, knees, and/or spine. Typically, such pain is worse following activity, and is relieved by a period of rest in the patient with osteoarthritis.

THE PHYSICAL EXAMINATION *should* reveal

- A patient in good general health; and
- With regard to the **locomotor system,** it *may* reveal
  - Bony swelling and deformity of the DIP (Heberden's nodes) and PIP (Bouchard's nodes) joints, with sparing of the metacarpophalangeal joints and wrists

CAUSES OF INFLAMMATORY POLYARTHRITIS

If you think that the patient does not have degenerative arthritis, but rather an inflammatory process involving the joints, what are the likely causes that should be considered?

- Rheumatoid arthritis (RA)
- Systemic lupus erythematosus (SLE)
- Psoriatic arthritis

How might you reasonably attempt to differentiate among these disorders on the basis of the HISTORY?

The **SYSTEMS REVIEW** might reveal, with regard to

1. Her General Health

- Systemic symptoms such as
  - Fever, fatigue, lassitude and weight loss—suggestive of both RA and SLE
  - (Bacterial infection, especially subacute bacterial endocarditis and gonococcal arthritis, would also need consideration.)

2. Her Skin, Hair, and Nails

- The presence of a rash—suggestive of
  - SLE
  - Psoriatic arthritis
  - (A drug reaction, serum sickness, bacterial endocarditis, and gonococcal arthritis, Henoch-Schönlein purpura, and sarcoidosis would also need to be considered.)

- Photosensitivity—suggestive of SLE
- Pigmentary changes—suggestive of SLE
- Loss of hair—suggestive of SLE
- Nail changes—suggestive of SLE or psoriasis

3. Her Gastrointestinal System

- Recurrent mouth ulcers—suggestive of SLE (and perhaps Crohn's disease)
- Dryness of the mouth and difficulty swallowing—suggestive of the sicca syndrome and rheumatoid arthritis
- (Diarrhea, possibly with blood and mucus in the stool—suggestive of Crohn's disease or ulcerative colitis)

4. Her Respiratory System

- Pleuritic chest pain—suggestive of SLE
- Cough and effort dyspnea—suggestive of sarcoidosis

5. Her Cardiovascular System

- Central chest pain compatible with pericarditis—suggestive of SLE
- Raynaud's phenomenon—suggestive of SLE or RA

6. Her Locomotor System

- A complaint of *stiffness* of the joints on awakening, which is relieved with activity—very suggestive of rheumatoid arthritis
- Muscle weakness and pain—suggestive of polymyositis

Might the pattern of joint involvement aid in the differential diagnosis?

- Yes, to an extent. Asymmetric involvement would favor psoriatic arthritis, as would involvement of the DIP joints.
- MP and PIP joint involvement is compatible with all three disorders. The more severe the involvement, the more likely that the disorder is rheumatoid arthritis.
- Sacroiliac pain might indicate psoriatic arthritis (and ankylosing spondylitis). Pain in the wrists, elbows, knees, and ankles would be compatible with both RA and SLE.

7. Her Eyes

- A scratchy, gritty sensation in the eyes, compatible with keratoconjunctivitis sicca—and suggestive of RA

8. Her Central Nervous System and Mental Status

- The occurrence of convulsions
- A change in personality, with hyper-irritability, or obsessional or paranoid reactions
- A change in consciousness, with drowsiness and confusion; or
- A frank organic psychosis

—all suggestive of SLE.

- Focal neurological signs, or a peripheral neuropathy—also suggestive of SLE

REVIEW OF HER PAST HISTORY or **PROBLEM LIST** might reveal

- Previous documentation of RA, SLE, or psoriasis, with obvious implications; or previous episodes of skin rash, pleuritic chest pain, pneumonia, pericarditis, a psychotic illness, neurologic disease, renal disease, a hemolytic anemia, or thrombocytopenia

—all *now* suggestive of SLE, in the context of her polyarthritis.

Her **FAMILY HISTORY** might reveal

- An established or suggestive diagnosis of SLE in other family members, which would support a diagnosis of SLE in the patient herself

Her **CURRENT LIFE SITUATION** might reveal

- Potential exposure to venereal disease—rendering a gonococcal arthritis possible

The **DRUG HISTORY** might reveal

- Administration of drugs likely to cause or exacerbate SLE— *e.g.,* hydralazine, isoniazid, phenytoin (Dilantin), procainamide, penicillin, sulfonamides, and the oral contraceptives

How might the PHYSICAL EXAMINATION aid the differential diagnostic process?

With regard to

1. The General Appearance

- An acutely ill, toxic-looking, febrile patient would suggest SLE, particularly; but a bacterial infection, especially subacute bacterial endocarditis, would need to be excluded in this circumstance.

2. Vital Signs

- Significant fever would suggest SLE or infection.
- Hypertension would suggest SLE.

3. The Skin and Nails

- *An erythematous rash* involving especially the face, neck, and fingertips would be very suggestive of SLE. More typical lesions comprise areas with fine scaling and follicular plugging. Areas of hyperpigmentation or vitiligo would also suggest SLE.
- *A petechial rash* might also suggest SLE; but Henoch-Schönlein purpura would need to be considered.
- *The characteristic erythrosquamous eruption of psoriasis* would obviously suggest psoriatic arthritis, more particularly if there were pitting of the nails, loosening and separation of the distal nail plate, or opaque, yellow areas of discoloration in the nail.
- *The presence of subcutaneous nodules,* especially over the olecranon process and the ulna, would be very suggestive of rheumatoid arthritis.
- *Erythema nodosum* would suggest sarcoidosis, or possibly a drug reaction. Papules, nodules, or plaques in the skin of the face, particularly, would also suggest sarcoidosis. The presence of facial and upper trunk erythema might also suggest dermatomyositis.
- *Thickening and tightening of the skin,* most prominently over the hands, would suggest scleroderma.

4. The Head and Neck

- Alopecia would be suggestive of SLE.
- Thickening and hyperemia of the bulbar conjunctivae would suggest keratoconjunctivitis sicca and RA. Retinal changes comprising "cotton wool" exudates (cytoid bodies) and hemorrhages would be very suggestive of SLE.

- The presence of cranial nerve palsies might suggest SLE; sarcoidosis also should be considered.
- An altered mental status and a psychotic illness would suggest SLE.
- Generalized lymphadenopathy would suggest SLE, particularly, but also RA and possibly sarcoidosis, or a lymphomatous process.

5. The Chest and Precordium

- A pleural rub or a pleural effusion would be very suggestive of SLE, as would a pericardial rub.

6. The Abdomen

- Splenomegaly would be suggestive of both SLE and RA. A lymphoma, SBE, and sarcoidosis would also need consideration.

7. The Extremities

- Symmetrical soft-tissue swelling of the proximal interphalangeal joints, with a consequent spindle-shaped appearance of the fingers, would be most suggestive of RA, but would be compatible with psoriatic arthritis.
- Asymmetrical DIP joint involvement would be more suggestive of psoriatic arthritis.
- The more florid the signs of inflammation in the MP and PIP joints, the more would RA be favored over SLE.
- The presence of a variety of neurologic abnormalities would suggest SLE, or possibly polyarteritis nodosa.
- A carpal tunnel syndrome might suggest RA.

What laboratory studies would be reasonable in the initial further investigation of this patient?

- Urinalysis
- Blood count, including hemoglobin, mean corpuscular volume, leukocyte count and differential, platelet count, reticulocyte count, erythrocyte sedimentation rate
- Protein electrophoresis
- Rheumatoid factor assay
- Antinuclear factor assay
- Radiographs of chest and affected joints

If you are still in doubt, what else is indicated?

- Careful observation at monthly intervals
- Consultation

EFFECTS OF POLYARTHRITIS

How might you assess the consequences or effects of this patient's arthritis?

It is necessary to determine the presence and extent of her *functional disability.*

This may be achieved from the **HISTORY** and **PHYSICAL EXAMINATION.**

The **HISTORY** relevant to the **CURRENT LIFE SITUATION** is most important in this regard. It is necessary to know how she is managing in her daily routine:

- Can she dress herself?
- Can she hold a knife and fork, a teacup, and feed herself?
- Can she manage on the toilet?
- Can she manage her housework and/or her job (what are her commitments in these areas)?
- Can she walk, and to what extent is walking limited?

From the **PHYSICAL EXAMINATION** it is possible to determine precisely which joints are involved, and the range of movement possible in each.

On the basis of the information elicited from the above approach, the diagnostic progression in this patient might have been from:

> Painful fingers
> ⟶ Polyarthritis
> ⟶ Rheumatoid arthritis

Determining the cause for rheumatoid arthritis is a research problem.

The potential effects of rheumatoid arthritis require careful assessment.

EFFECTS OF RHEUMATOID ARTHRITIS

What are the consequences of rheumatoid arthritis (RA)?

- The additive involvement of other joints

- The development of joint deformities
- The development of extra-articular manifestations of the disease
- Complications of therapy
- The coincidental development of other diseases commonly associated with rheumatoid arthritis

While many extra-articular manifestations of RA have been described, only a few are relatively common—which?

- Those involving the *eye*
  - Keratoconjunctivitis sicca (KS)
  - Scleritis and its complications
- Those involving the *extremities*
  - Rheumatoid nodules
  - Vasculitis
  - Carpal tunnel syndrome
- Those involving the *hemopoietic system*
  - Anemia
  - Felty's syndrome

How might you detect the development of these disorders?

The **SYSTEMS REVIEW** might reveal, with regard to

1. Eye, Ear, Nose, and Throat

- Burning or smarting of the eyes, a gritty sensation in the eyes; and/or dryness of the mouth, with difficulty swallowing—suggestive of keratoconjunctivitis sicca
- A complaint of deep ocular pain and/or a disturbance of vision—suggestive of scleritis
- Complaints of redness of the eye, or photophobia, compatible with both KS and scleritis

2. The Cardiovascular System

- Painful extremities, sometimes with digital ulceration—suggestive of vasculitis

3. The Nervous System

- Paraesthesias in the hands, especially at night, suggestive of the carpal tunnel syndrome. (Sometimes, but often not, this may be localized to the distribution of the median nerve.)

The **PHYSICAL EXAMINATION** might reveal, with regard to

1. **The Eyes**

   - A yellowish white, thick, tenacious secretion at the inner corner of the eyelids; tenacious mucus strands in the lower conjunctival fornix; and/or thickening and hyperemia of the bulbar conjunctivae—all suggestive of keratoconjunctivitis sicca
   - A localized area of hyperemia in the sclera, sometimes associated with the presence of a small nodule—suggestive of episcleritis
   - Thinning of the sclera, such that the bluish black discoloration of the uvea is evident—suggestive of more significant scleritis or pending scleromalacia perforans

2. **The Abdomen**

   - Splenomegaly, suggestive of (among other conditions) Felty's syndrome

3. **The Extremities**

   - Subcutaneous nodules over the olecranon process and along the ulnar surface of the forearms—indicative of rheumatoid nodules
   - Small brown areas in the nail fold, nail edge, or digital pulp —suggestive of rheumatoid vasculitis
   - Loss of sensation over the palmar aspects of the thumb, index, middle and radial aspects of the ring fingers, wasting of the thenar muscles, and weakness of opposition—strongly indicative of carpal tunnel syndrome

What laboratory or further studies are indicated?

- Full blood count to detect anemia, the neutropenia of Felty's syndrome, and the hematologic effects of drug therapy
- Fluorescein staining of the cornea and a labial biopsy to confirm KS, if it is suspected on the basis of either the history or the physical examination, and perhaps even as a routine test in such patients in the absence of clinical clues

- Nerve conduction studies, if indicated by a clinical suspicion of carpal tunnel syndrome

What other disorders are likely to be associated with RA?

Empirical observation has indicated that RA is associated with the following disorders in a frequency greater than that in the general population:

- Diabetes mellitus
- Hypothyroidism
- Pernicious anemia

It is thus well to keep these possibilities in mind when following a patient with rheumatoid arthritis.

ACUTE ARTHRITIS IN A SINGLE LARGE JOINT

During your rotation in the emergency ward you see a 42-year-old man who complains that he has had increasing pain and swelling in his left knee over the past 12 hours.

On physical examination you note that the knee is slightly flexed.

Further inspection reveals a horseshoe-shaped fullness above the knee and around its medial and lateral margins.

Both passive and active movements are exquisitely painful, and the patient both resents and resists these.

The knee is warm to the touch and tender, and "fluctuation" of the joint can be detected.

How would you formulate this clinical problem?

As "acute arthritis of the left knee."

What are likely possibilities that would account for this?

- Trauma
- Sepsis
- Gout
- A hemarthrosis due to a bleeding diathesis
- Rheumatoid arthritis
- Reiter's syndrome

How might you attempt to differentiate between these disorders—on the basis of the HISTORY?

With regard to

1. The Present Circumstances

- Recent injury to the knee would obviously be very suggestive of trauma as the cause for a painful effusion. However, the details of the incident should be carefully elicited, since this could be a "red herring."

2. The Systems Review, relevant to

- **His general health**
  - ○ Fever, and other systemic symptoms such as fatigue, malaise, and lassitude, would be very suggestive of a septic arthritis.
  - ○ (A low-grade fever would also be compatible with acute gouty arthritis, possibly rheumatoid arthritis, and Reiter's syndrome.)
- **His eyes, ears, nose, and throat**
  - ○ A complaint of a "red eye," associated with early-morning stickiness of the eyelids, and a conjunctival discharge—features indicative of conjunctivitis—would be very suggestive of Reiter's syndrome. Lesser symptoms might also suggest RA.
- **His genitourinary system**
  - ○ Complaints of dysuria, frequency and a urethral discharge would be suggestive of both Reiter's syndrome and gonococcal arthritis.
  - ○ Ulceration of the glans penis would be suggestive of Reiter's syndrome.
- **His locomotor system**
  - ○ Pain in other joints as well would be suggestive of Reiter's syndrome, gonococcal and other septic arthritides, and rheumatoid arthritis.
  - ○ Morning stiffness would be suggestive of RA.
- **His gastrointestinal system**
  - ○ Painful mouth ulcers would be suggestive of Reiter's syndrome.
- **His skin**
  - ○ Painful skin lesions on the soles of his feet would be suggestive of Reiter's syndrome.

3. The Problem List and/or Past History

- A known diagnosis of
  - Hemophilia
  - Gout, or
  - Rheumatoid arthritis

would have obvious, but not definitive, diagnostic implications.

- Previous isolated or recurrent episodes of trauma to the knee would imply a traumatic basis.
- Previous episodes of conjunctivitis or urethritis would be suggestive of Reiter's syndrome, or possibly gonococcal arthritis.
- Previous episodes of arthritis in other joints would be suggestive of *gout,* if in the tarso-metatarsal joints; of *hemophilia,* if several other large joints; of RA, if small joints of the hands, had been involved.
- Abnormal bleeding in the past would be suggestive of a hemarthrosis.

4. The Family History

- A diagnosis of gout or hemophilia in other family members would have obvious implications.

5. The Current Life Situation

- Participation in vigorous sporting activities would make a traumatic process more likely, even if no specific incident could be recalled.
- Appropriate sexual exposure would suggest a gonococcal arthritis.

6. The Drug History

- Anticoagulant ingestion would suggest an acute hemarthrosis

How might the PHYSICAL EXAMINATION aid the diagnostic process?

It might reveal, with regard to

1. His General Appearance

- A toxic-looking, ill subject—suggestive of a septic process

2. The Vital Signs

- Pyrexia—suggestive of a septic arthritis, but also of Reiter's syndrome and possibly RA or gout

3. The Head and Neck

- Conjunctival redness and discharge, suggestive of Reiter's syndrome
- Gouty tophi on the ear, suggestive of acute gouty arthritis
- Mouth ulcers, suggestive of Reiter's syndrome

4. The External Genitalia

- A urethral discharge, suggestive of gonococcal arthritis and Reiter's syndrome
- Ulcers around the glans, suggestive of Reiter's syndrome

5. The Extremities and Back

- Painless limitation of movement of other joints—suggestive of hemophilia
- Painful involvement of other joints, compatible with sepsis, gout, RA, or Reiter's syndrome
- Tenderness over the sacroiliac joints—suggestive of rheumatoid arthritis and Reiter's syndrome
- Olecranon bursitis—suggestive of gout
- Rheumatoid nodules—suggestive of RA
- Keratoderma blenorrhagica—suggestive of Reiter's syndrome

What investigations are indicated?

These will depend upon your clinical suspicions. If there were the least possibility of a septic arthritis—irrespective of other diagnostic considerations, *aspiration of the joint,* with detailed examination of the aspirate, should be performed.

If a diagnosis of septic arthritis were confirmed in this patient, the diagnostic progression would have been from

> A painful swollen knee
> ⟶ Acute arthritis
> ⟶ Acute septic arthritis

The questions now to be posed are:

- Why does this patient have a septic arthritis?
- What are its possible consequences, and are any evident?

Knowledge as to likely causes and effects, and their clinical manifestations is again required. The orderly history and physical examination can, as always, be used as a means of discovering the clinical clues that will help you to answer these questions.

CHAPTER 9

Easy Bruising

A frequent complaint by patients is that they "bruise easily," or that they are "bleeders."

Such a complaint demands a decision as to whether the patient is indeed abnormal, and whether he does, or does not, have a significant bleeding disorder.

If not, further investigation is obviously inappropriate, the prognosis is excellent, and surgery, if necessary, can be safely advocated.

Conversely, if the patient does have a bleeding disorder, its cause and mechanism must then be established, since prognosis and treatment will be dictated by these factors.

As an intern in surgery, while interviewing a 32-year-old female patient who is due for elective surgery the following day, you learn that she is a "bleeder, you know."

CLINICAL FEATURES OF A BLEEDING DIATHESIS

How might you attempt to decide whether or not she has a significant bleeding disorder?

By determining whether

- There is clinical evidence of abnormal bleeding
- The clinical circumstances are such that abnormal bleeding is probable, and therefore to be anticipated
- There is laboratory evidence of a bleeding tendency

What would constitute "clinical evidence of abnormal bleeding"?

- "Spontaneous" bleeding
- Prolonged or excessive bleeding following trauma; and/or
- Bleeding from several different sites

What "clinical circumstances" in this patient would enhance the likelihood that a bleeding disorder is present?

If there were a *well-substantiated* history of abnormal bleeding in other family members, this would be very suggestive of a possible INHERITED BLEEDING DISORDER.

An ACQUIRED BLEEDING DISORDER would be suspect in the face of certain disease entities, more particularly

- Liver disease
- Renal disease, and
- Malignant disease

and in association with the administration of drugs such as

- Aspirin
- Sodium warfarin, or
- Heparin

How might you detect the presence of abnormal bleeding, or the circumstances indicating a potential bleeding diathesis?

THE HISTORY is especially useful in this regard.

THE REVIEW OF SYSTEMS might reveal evidence of bleeding from a number of sites.

If the extent and frequency of such bleeding were "abnormal," this would imply a significant disorder.

Thus, it is important to know about the *existence of,* and then the onset, course, duration, character, severity, aggravating and precipitating factors of the following symptoms in

1. The Eyes, Ears, Nose, and Throat

- Nose bleeds
- Bleeding from the gums

2. The Gastrointestinal Tract

- Hematemesis
- Melena
- The passage of fresh blood per rectum

3. The Respiratory Tract

- Hemoptysis

4. The Genitourinary Tract

- Hematuria
- Vaginal bleeding

5. The Skin

- Bruising
- Hematoma formation
- A petechial rash

A **REVIEW OF THE PROBLEM LIST** or the **PAST HIS-TORY** might reveal evidence of

1. **Excessive or Prolonged Bleeding.** Such bleeding might be related to

- Trauma
- Surgical procedures, or
- Dental procedures

This would obviously increase the likelihood that a significant bleeding disorder is present; while previous major trauma without abnormal bleeding, would, conversely, be quite reassuring, at least as to the absence of a significant *inherited* disorder. Exceptions exist, however, and a number of hemophiliac infants have been circumcised without difficulty.

The extent of the putative abnormal bleeding must be assessed. This can be done by determining the duration of prior hospitalizations and/or the need for blood transfusion. If necessary, hospital records and the physicians concerned should be consulted, since patients' descriptions of such matters are peculiarly liable to distortion.

2. Prior Documentation of Liver, Renal, or Malignant Disease

A review of the **FAMILY HISTORY** might reveal

- The existence of abnormal bleeding in other family members

A review of **MEDICATIONS** is clearly indicated—with a careful search for aspirin or anticoagulant ingestion as a major objective.

What features on PHYSICAL EXAMINATION would support the presence of a bleeding diathesis?

- Signs of abnormal bleeding
- Evidence of chronic blood loss
- Signs of those disorders known to be associated with bleeding disorders

What are the signs of abnormal bleeding?

These include, with regard to the

- Skin
  - Extensive bruising
  - Hematomas
  - A petechial rash
- Musculoskeletal system
  - Ankylosis of joints

In a postoperative patient it would also be useful to inspect

- The nasogastric aspirate
- The urinary catheter
- Venipuncture sites
- Intramuscular injection sites
- The operative wound
- Drainage sites

What are the signs of chronic blood loss?

These are essentially the signs of iron deficiency, and are seen in the

- Hand
  - Brittle, broken nails
  - Thin nails
  - Koilonychia
- Eye
  - Pallor of the conjunctivae
  - Blue discoloration of the sclerae
- Mouth
  - Angular stomatitis
  - Pallor of the mucous membranes
  - Atrophic glossitis
- Abdomen
  - Occasionally, splenomegaly

What underlying disease manifestations would you look for?

The features of

- Liver disease—discussed in Chapter 16
- Renal disease—Chapter 7
- Malignant disease—Chapter 2

What laboratory studies are routinely indicated in the investigation of a patient with a suspected bleeding disorder?

- A platelet count
- A bleeding time—only in the adult, and only if the platelet count is *normal*
- Prothrombin time, partial thromboplastin time, and thrombin time determinations
- A complete blood count
- Assays of the serum BUN, creatinine, SGOT, alkaline phosphatase, and total protein concentrations

The final judgment as to the presence of a bleeding disorder will depend on a careful analysis of *all* of the information obtained above.

Clinical evidence of abnormal bleeding should never be discarded in the face of normal laboratory screening tests, and always demands attention.

Should abnormal bleeding be substantiated, the next step in the diagnostic process will be to try to establish both its mechanism and its cause.

This requires knowledge of the potential mechanisms for abnormal bleeding, and the more likely causes.

MECHANISMS OF ABNORMAL BLEEDING

What are the mechanisms that might be responsible for a bleeding disorder?

DEFECTIVE HEMOSTASIS, due to

- Platelet abnormalities
  - Thrombocytopenia
  - Dysfunctional platelets
- Vascular abnormalities
- Defects of the extravascular supporting structures

DEFECTIVE COAGULATION, due to

- Diminished production
- Inhibition of function
- Destruction, or
- Loss

—of one or several of the different coagulation factors

CAUSES OF ABNORMAL BLEEDING

What are the likely causes of a bleeding diathesis?

INHERITED DISEASE, especially

- Hemophilia
- Von Willebrand's disease
- Christmas disease
- A platelet functional disorder

ACQUIRED DISEASE

- Liver disease
- Renal disease
- Malignant disease
- Infection
- The effects of drug therapy
- Obstetrical complications

How might you proceed in order to try to determine the mechanism, and the cause, of the abnormal bleeding in a particular patient?

Initially, by considering those suggested by the

- Specific clinical circumstances
- Clinical findings, and/or
- Laboratory findings

in *that* patient; and then by utilizing further clinical or laboratory investigations to exclude or confirm the various postulates.

On further evaluation of the 32-year-old female patient described previously, you learn that she has "always bruised easily," with minimal trauma and often spontaneously, and that cuts seem to continue bleeding for an excessively long period of time.

Her menstrual flow is "heavy," and associated with the passage of clots. Dysmenorrhea is a problem.

Two dental extractions were complicated by persistent oozing for 2 to 3 days.

Her mother "bruises easily."

Her template bleeding time is 18 minutes. Other screening tests are normal.

What disorders are suggested in this patient?

The symptoms are fairly typical of defective hemostasis, as opposed to defective coagulation.

- *Thrombocytopenia* would need consideration, but is excluded by a normal platelet count.
- *A dysfunctional platelet disorder* is quite probable.

The potentially positive family history suggests an inherited disorder, while the dysmenorrhea indicates probable analgesic use—particularly aspirin—which might well explain an acquired platelet dysfunction. (A patient who takes aspirin only once or twice a month with her dysmenorrhea will probably deny use of analgesics on casual questioning.)

The prolongation of the bleeding time, as an isolated finding, certainly supports a diagnosis of defective hemostasis as a result of platelet dysfunction.

Von Willebrand's disease also needs careful consideration because of both the symptomatology and the prolongation of the bleeding time.

Further differentiation between these two possibilities will require sophisticated laboratory investigation.

OTHER ILLUSTRATIVE CASE STUDIES

An 18-year-old man is admitted to the hospital for elective tonsillectomy. He has no history of abnormal bleeding. His partial thromboplastin time (PTT) is markedly prolonged at 102 sec (control, 36 sec). There are no other abnormal laboratory findings.

What disorders are suggested in this patient?

Prolongation of the PTT as a totally isolated finding, in the absence of a history of abnormal bleeding, is very suggestive of

- Factor XII deficiency

Caution would nevertheless dictate that

- Deficiencies of factors VIII and IX and
- The presence of a circulating anticoagulant

be excluded. Specific laboratory studies can be directed to differentiating between these possibilities.

A 36-year-old female patient is admitted to the hematology ward because of the sudden onset of abnormal bleeding. She has developed bleeding from her gums, extensive bruising, hematuria, and epistaxis.

She was well until 2 days previously, when she noted the sudden onset of right flank pain, chills, fever, and hematuria.

She has had four pregnancies, none of which was associated with excessive blood loss, and she has not bled excessively after tooth extraction or following tonsillectomy or appendectomy. There is no family history of abnormal bleeding.

She sought medical attention 2 years previously, following the sudden onset of left-sided weakness. Mitral stenosis with cerebral embolism was diagnosed, and she was treated with bishydroxycoumarin.

After 6 and 9 months she experienced severe episodes of vaginal bleeding, each requiring blood transfusion, and the oral anticoagulant was discontinued.

Physical examination reveals bleeding from the gums and extensive bruising. A large hematoma is present at the site of an intramuscular injection. Venipuncture is followed by persistent oozing.

Abdominal examination reveals a 26-week pregnancy.

Prothrombin time determined prior to her referral was 64 sec (control, 12 sec).

What disorders are suggested by this constellation of findings?

The negative past history and family history largely exclude an *inherited* disorder, and the sudden onset further supports the probability of an *acquired* bleeding disorder.

- The history of flank pain, hematuria, fever, and chills is very suggestive of a urinary tract infection, and possible consequent *septicemia.*
- This in turn strongly suggests that the acquired bleeding disorder in this patient might be a result of
  - Disseminated intravascular coagulation (DIC), or possibly
  - Thrombocytopenia per se
- *Pregnancy,* in association with an acquired bleeding disorder, must suggest the possibility of an *abruptio placentae*— with consequent disseminated intravascular coagulation.
- The possibility that she might have attempted to induce an *abortion,* and that *septicemia* and *DIC* might be consequences of this, also needs consideration.
- Valvular heart disease and fever must raise the suspicion of *bacterial endocarditis;* again, DIC and thrombocytopenia should be considered.
- Prior exposure, and access to, oral anticoagulants must at

least suggest the possibility of an acquired bleeding diathesis on this basis.

- The prolongation of the prothrombin time is, per se, confirmatory of defective coagulation. The potential mechanisms suggested by the clinical picture in this patient are:
  - *Destruction of coagulation factors* in the course of disseminated intravascular coagulation, and possibly
  - *Defective production of coagulation factors*, resulting from the ingestion of oral anticoagulants

Further considerations to explain a prolongation of the prothrombin time would include:

- Defective production of coagulation factors, due to
  - Liver disease, or
  - A vitamin K deficiency state

resulting from either dietary lack, or malabsorption.

(An inherited defect of one of the coagulation proteins of the extrinsic pathway is essentially excluded by the history, in this patient.)

How should you proceed?

- To laboratory tests aimed at confirming or excluding disseminated intravascular coagulation.
- To laboratory tests aimed at considering the possibility of oral anticoagulant ingestion.
- To clinical and laboratory investigations that will confirm or exclude
  - A urinary tract infection
  - Bacterial endocarditis
  - Septicemia, or
  - Abruptio placentae
- Possibly to clinical and laboratory investigations that will confirm or exclude a dietary deficiency, a malabsorption state, and liver disease

A 64-year-old chronic alcoholic, with cirrhosis of the liver, is admitted for bleeding esophageal varices, and will probably require surgery. Prior to such surgery, help is requested in assessing and managing a possible bleeding diathesis.

What mechanisms might account for abnormal bleeding in a patient with chronic liver disease and chronic alcoholism?

Liver disease and chronic alcoholism can result in an acquired bleeding diathesis through virtually every conceivable mechanism. Thus **defective hemostasis** can result from

- *Thrombocytopenia,* due to
  - Congestive splenomegaly
  - A folate-deficient diet
  - The myelosuppressive effects of alcohol
  - Massive blood loss
  - Septicemia
- Dysfunctional platelets, due to increased level of fibrinogen and fibrin degradation products.

Abnormalities of the coagulation mechanism can result from

- A decreased synthesis of coagulation factors, due to
  - Hepatocellular dysfunction, and
  - Malabsorption of vitamin K
- The presence of circulating anticoagulants (fibrinogen or fibrin degradation products), due to the increased fibrinolysis which occurs in liver disease for a variety of reasons
- Increased destruction of coagulation factors, due to disseminated intravascular coagulation or increased fibrinolysis
- "Washout" of coagulation factors, following, for example, massive variceal bleeding. This is always quite apparent clinically.

How should you proceed?

Laboratory investigations can contribute quite significantly to the documentation of the more predominant mechanisms in a particular patient.

Appropriate therapy—pre-, intra-, and post-operative—can then be instituted.

In a patient with a possible bleeding diathesis, this diagnosis should be established as firmly as possible. The mechanisms and the cause can usually be suspected from a careful evaluation of the clinical findings, the known clinical circumstances, and routine laboratory studies, and can be confirmed with more specific investigations.

CHAPTER 10

Headache

Headache is a common symptom. In the majority of instances, it is self-treated with some form of patent medicine.

The problem for the physician is to know when to pursue it further, and the extent to which headache in a particular patient should be investigated. This is especially difficult when the symptom is elicited in the course of a routine systems review:

STUDENT: "Are you troubled with headaches?"
PATIENT: "Oh yes!—sometimes."

The decision must depend upon either

- The likelihood that the headache reflects significant disease
- The extent to which it is bothering, or incapacitating, the patient

ACUTE HEADACHE

While you are in the emergency department, you are asked to evaluate a 45-year-old woman who complains of the sudden onset of headache.

Should this problem be pursued further?

Here the answer is easy. If the patient herself is seeking help for the problem, it must be pursued. Furthermore, the fact that she has come to the emergency room should in itself alert you to the possibility that there may be a serious causative process, possibly requiring urgent diagnosis and management.

113

In what disorders is headache a prominent symptom that demands urgent assessment and perhaps even "invasive" investigation?

- Meningitis
- A rapidly expanding subdural or extradural hematoma
- Hypertensive encephalopathy
- A subarachnoid hemorrhage
- Hypoglycemia
- Carbon monoxide poisoning
- Acute glaucoma
- A cerebrovascular accident

What features in the history will heighten the probability of one or another of these "urgent" disorders?

A more detailed **ANALYSIS OF THE HEADACHE** per se might reveal, with regard to its

1. Onset

- A sudden, explosive onset—very suggestive of a subarachnoid hemorrhage

2. Site and Radiation

- Pain felt initially in the eyeball and homolateral frontal region—possibly suggestive of glaucoma, a berry aneurysm, or a diabetic neuropathy
- Pain in the occiput, radiating into the neck and spine—suggestive of meningitis or a subarachnoid hemorrhage

3. Severity

- Very severe pain, certainly suggestive of serious or urgent disease

The **REVIEW OF SYSTEMS** might reveal, with regard to

1. Her General Health

- Fever—suggestive of meningitis
- Sweating—perhaps suggestive of hypoglycemia

2. The Central Nervous System

- Drowsiness

- Convulsions, and/or
- Focal neurologic symptoms

—all highly indicative of serious pathology.

3. The Eyes

- Diplopia—very suggestive of an expanding aneurysm and/or a subarachnoid hemorrhage, particularly
- Photophobia—suggestive of meningitis, a subarachnoid hemorrhage, and perhaps glaucoma
- Blurring of vision or "iridescent haloes" seen around lights —symptoms suggestive of glaucoma

A review of the **PROBLEM LIST or PAST HISTORY** might reveal information that would render some of these disorders more probable. For example:

- Known ear or sinus infection
- A previous skull fracture
- Previous neurosurgical intervention, or
- An immunocompromised state

would very much increase the likelihood of meningitis.

- A known diabetic
- A known alcoholic
- A patient with adrenocortical insufficiency, or a functioning pancreatic islet cell tumor

would be very likely to develop hypoglycemia.

- A known hypertensive subject
- A patient with a documented pheochromocytoma, or
- A patient with renal disease

would be at increased risk for hypertensive encephalopathy, or a cerebrovascular accident.

- A history of recent *trauma* would very much increase the likelihood of a rapidly expanding subdural, or extradural, hematoma.
- Previous documentation of any of the disorders would certainly raise the suspicion of its recurrence.

A review of the **LIFE SITUATION** might reveal, for example:

- Lower socioeconomic status, or recent camping or mountaineering and the exposure in these circumstances to a coal-burning brazier, which would increase the suspicion of carbon monoxide poisoning.

What features in the PHYSICAL EXAMINATION might be significant clues to urgent pathology?

With regard to

1. **Her General Appearance**

   - An "acutely ill" patient, lying curled up, might have meningitis.
   - The patient who lies very still is likely to have a subarachnoid hemorrhage.

2. **The Vital Signs**

   - Pyrexia would be suggestive of meningitis.
   - Marked hypertension would be very suggestive of hypertensive encephalopathy, a subarachnoid hemorrhage, or an intracerebral hemorrhage.

3. **The Mental Status**

   - Drowsiness, stupor, or coma would all be highly indicative of urgent disease.
   - Similarly, irritability, restlessness, difficulty with speech or thought, agitation or confusion, would also all be important clues to urgent disease.

4. **The Head.** Examination might reveal in the

   - Scalp
     - Signs of trauma, suggestive of an intracranial hematoma
   - Eye
     - Conjunctival redness, and/or tenderness of the eyeball—suggestive of acute glaucoma
     - Fundal changes: (1) Hypertensive changes suggestive of hypertensive encephalopathy, or an intracerebral hemorrhage. (2) Papilledema, suggestive of hypertensive encephalopathy, meningitis, or an expanding hematoma. (3) Subhyaloid hemorrhages, suggestive of a subarachnoid hemorrhage. (4) Diabetic retinopathy, perhaps suggestive of hypoglycemia

- ○ Evidence of a third nerve palsy—very suggestive of an aneurysm, and hence of a subarachnoid hemorrhage; or of a diabetic neuropathy
- Mouth
  - ○ A cherry red discoloration of the buccal mucosa—very suggestive of carbon monoxide poisoning
- Ears and sinuses
  - ○ Middle ear conduction deafness or a purulent discharge from the ear; or
  - ○ Tenderness over the mastoid, frontal, or maxillary sinuses

features suggestive of the possibility of superimposed meningitis.

5. The Neck

- *Neck stiffness,* and/or
- A positive Brudzinski's sign

—which would be very strongly indicative of either meningitis or a subarachnoid hemorrhage.

6. The Extremities

- Focal neurologic signs—suggestive of an intracranial hemorrhage or other cerebrovascular accident, hypertensive encephalopathy, and also of meningitis and perhaps hypoglycemia
- Kernig's sign—very suggestive of a subarachnoid hemorrhage, or of meningitis

Are laboratory investigations indicated?

This will very much depend upon the findings elicited from the history and examination.

- If there is any suspicion of meningitis, *lumbar puncture* is indicated.
- Similarly, the possibility of a subarachnoid hemorrhage should also be pursued with a *lumbar puncture.*

Extreme caution is indicated, however, in the patient with lateralizing signs, and/or raised intracranial pressure, or in whom an intracranial hematoma is suspected. In such patients, computerized axial tomography of the brain, and a specialist's opinion, are essential before proceeding.

- Hypoglycemia can be readily excluded or confirmed with a blood glucose determination, and, if suspected, should be treated immediately and without awaiting the results of the assay.
- Carbon monoxide poisoning can be confirmed biochemically or spectrophotometrically, and if suspected should also be treated prior to confirmation.
- Acute glaucoma can be confirmed by measuring intraocular tension.

What other disorders presenting with headache provoking a visit to the emergency room should you consider?

- Systemic infections
- Any of the disorders that can cause *recurrent headaches* (and that are considered in a subsequent section of this chapter)

What clinical symptoms and signs would suggest a systemic infection as the cause for this patient's headache?

In the **REVIEW OF SYSTEMS,** relevant to

1. **Her General Health**
   - Fever, chills, rigors, and sweating
   - Malaise, lassitude, and fatigue

2. **The Gastrointestinal System**
   - Anorexia, nausea, vomiting, diarrhea, or constipation

3. **The Eyes, Ears, Nose, and Throat**
   - Rhinorrhea
   - Sore throat
   - Hoarseness

4. **The Respiratory System**
   - Cough

5. **The Musculoskeletal System**
   - Myalgia
   - Arthralgia
6. **The Genitourinary System**
   - Frequency
   - Dysuria
7. **The Skin**
   - Rashes

In the **PHYSICAL EXAMINATION,** with regard to

1. **Her General Appearance**
   - A toxic appearance
2. **The Vital Signs**
   - Pyrexia
   - Tachycardia
   - Tachypnea
   - Hypotension
3. **Her Mental Status**
   - Delirium
4. **Her Head and Neck**
   - Conjunctival injection
   - Rhinorrhea
   - Pharyngitis
   - Lymphadenopathy
5. **The Abdomen**
   - Splenomegaly
6. **The Skin**
   - A rash
   - Warm, dry skin
7. **The Extremities**
   - Muscle tenderness

RECURRENT HEADACHES

During your rotation in the family medicine department, you are asked to evaluate a 55-year-old female patient whose reason for coming to the clinic is "frequent headaches."

What, in order of probability, are the disorders that are most likely to explain this patient's headaches?

- Tension headaches
- Migraine
- Disorders of the nose, ears, eyes, teeth, and sinuses

What less likely, but potentially serious disorders, with significant prognostic and therapeutic implications, should you also consider?

- Hypertension
- Temporal arteritis
- The various consequences of alcohol excess
- The various consequences of trauma
- "Intracranial mass lesions"—such as brain tumor, brain abscess, or subdural hematoma

Are the "urgent" disorders discussed above excluded?

It is wise to remember that a subarachnoid hemorrhage, hypoglycemia, glaucoma, and carbon monoxide poisoning could be recurrent.

How might you utilize the HISTORY to help you differentiate among these various disorders?

A DESCRIPTION OF THE CHARACTERISTICS OF THE HEADACHE is usually helpful, and may well be diagnostic. Thus, with regard to its

1. Onset

The *recent* occurrence of headaches increases the suspicion of

- A mass lesion

- Disorders of local structures
- Hypertension, and
- Temporal arteritis

Conversely, a *long-standing* history of recurrent headaches is more suggestive of migraine or tension headaches.

2. Time of Occurrence

- The presence of pain on awakening in the morning suggests hypertension, migraine, or glaucoma.
- Pain coming on in the early part of the day suggests nasal or paranasal sinus disease, or possibly brain tumor.
- Pain occurring in the latter part of the day suggests muscle tension headache or disorders of the eye.
- Pain occurring repeatedly between midnight and 2 A.M. is suggestive of cluster headaches.

3. Duration

- Pain lasting a few hours suggests cluster headaches, brain tumor, "disease of local structures," or hypertension. Migraine is also self-limited, lasting 8–12 hours or less, but may blend into a muscle tension headache lasting for several days.
- Pain lasting for several days is usually due to a tension headache.
- Sharp, lancinating pain lasting seconds suggests a neuralgia.

4. Course

- Attacks of pain recurring at intervals of weeks or months suggest migraine.
- Pain occurring daily, for days or weeks on end, followed by a long period with no pain, suggests cluster headaches.
- Pain of recent onset, recurring several times a day, especially if of increasing frequency and severity and with a background of minimal or no headache, is very worrisome with regard to a mass lesion.
- Daily pain also suggests hypertension, muscle tension headache, sinus, eye, or other "local" disease.

5. Site

- Pain in the *temporal regions* is perhaps more likely to be due to migraine, cranial arteritis, or a cluster headache.

- *Occipital headaches* are likely to result from tension headaches or hypertension, but could also be caused by diseases of the eye, cervical spine, or posterior fossa tumors.
- *Orbital pain,* frontal pain, and pain over the vertex is likely to be due to "local" disease or a cluster headache but could reflect a mass lesion.
- *Facial pain* might be due to trigeminal neuralgia.
- *Throat and pharyngeal pain* might be due to glossopharyngeal neuralgia.

6. Character

- A throbbing pain usually suggests migraine, or arterial hypertension.
- A steady, aching pain suggests a mass lesion, "local" disease, arteritis, or tension headache. The latter often has a bandlike quality.

7. Severity

- A very severe pain suggests migraine, cluster headaches, neuralgia, a subdural hematoma, or glaucoma.
- More moderate pain could also result from these conditions, but would be more likely to result from tension headaches, hypertension, mass lesions, local disease, and temporal arteritis. (Seventy percent of tumors are *painless*.)

8. Aggravating and Relieving Factors

- Posture
  - Pain exacerbated by lying down, and relieved in the erect position, is suggestive of migraine, and of paranasal disease.
  - Headache that is worse in the erect position suggests a a mass lesion.
  - Stooping, or the head-down position, will aggravate most "headaches."

- Movement
  - Sudden movement, straining, or coughing will aggravate the pain of migraine, hypertension, sinusitis, or mass lesions.
  - Head jolt will aggravate the pain of migraine and intracranial masses.
  - The pain due to muscle tension is *not* affected by posture,

straining, or activity, but may be worsened by fatigue, anxiety, and depression.

○ Pressure on the superficial scalp arteries will often relieve the headache of migraine and of arterial hypertension.

The **REVIEW OF SYSTEMS** might be useful. With regard to

1. **Her General Health**

   • *Fever* would suggest sinusitis, otitis media, mastoiditis, or dental abscess; also, temporal arteritis.

   • *Loss of weight* and malaise would suggest temporal arteritis, or malignant disease with cerebral metastases.

2. **The Central Nervous System**

   • Hemi-sensory or motor deficits preceding the headache, or associated with it, would render migraine highly probable.

   • Focal symptoms that are persistent and outlast the headache would be indicative of a mass lesion.

3. **The Eyes, Ears, Nose, and Throat**

   • A variety of visual phenomena may precede an attack of migraine.

   • The sudden development of blindness would suggest temporal arteritis.

   • Visual field defects, or diplopia, might be indicative of a mass lesion.

   • Blurring of vision, and iridescent haloes on looking at lights would suggest glaucoma.

   • Earache, an aural discharge, or deafness would suggest a middle ear infection.

   • A nasal discharge, a postnasal drip, a sore throat, hoarseness, or cough would suggest paranasal infection.

   • Toothache, or pain on chewing would suggest dental or temporomandibular disease.

4. **The Musculoskeletal System**

   • Pain in the shoulders or hips would suggest the temporal arteritis/polymyalgia rheumatica complex.

A review of the **PAST HISTORY** or **PROBLEM LIST** might prove invaluable; for example:

   • A lifelong history of similar headaches would suggest migraine or tension headaches.

- Headache following trauma to the head would suggest
  - Postconcussion headaches
  - Subdural hematoma
  - Post-traumatic migraine
  - Tension headaches
  - Spinal column pathology
- A patient with known oat cell carcinoma of the lung who develops such recurrent headaches would be especially likely to have
  - Metastatic brain tumor
  - Meningeal infiltration by tumor
  - Tension headache
  - Post-lumbar-puncture headache
  - Systemic infection
- A patient with long-standing lung infections or with chronic ear or sinus infection might now have
  - A brain abscess

A review of her **LIFE SITUATION** might reveal

- Occupational, financial, or domestic circumstances likely to produce tension headaches
- Possible exposure to coal-burning braziers—and hence carbon monoxide poisoning
- Alcohol excesses, with its several implications
  - An increased likelihood of head trauma
  - Hypoglycemia
  - A hangover

A review of the **FAMILY HISTORY** might reveal evidence of

- Migraine or
- Hypertension

in other family members, with the obvious implications.

A review of the **DRUG HISTORY** might reveal that the patient is taking (for example):

- Monoamine oxidase inhibitors, or
- Amyl nitrite or nitroglycerine

—drugs that could be responsible for her headache.

How might the PHYSICAL EXAMINATION assist in the diagnosis?

With regard to

1. The Mental Status

- An altered mental status—change in personality, change in behavior patterns, alteration in intellectual functioning, judgement, etc.—would be very suggestive of a mass lesion.

2. The Vital Signs

- Hypertension per se might be the basis for her frequent headaches.
- Pyrexia would suggest an infectious cause—either local, or possibly systemic.

3. The Head and Neck

- Examination of the ears, nose, sinuses, and teeth might reveal evidence of infection that might account for her headaches.
- Fundal examination might reveal features of hypertensive disease, or of papilledema, which would very much suggest a mass lesion.
- Tenderness of the scalp and tenderness and/or thickening of the temporal arteries would suggest arteritis.
- Cranial nerve palsies would be very suggestive of a mass lesion.
- Limitation of neck movements might be indicative of cervical spine disease.

4. The Precordium

- Signs of hypertensive disease (*q.v.*) might be evident.

5. The Extremities

- Focal neurologic signs would strongly suggest a mass lesion.

What laboratory studies are indicated?

These will be very much determined by the findings and the diagnostic impressions gained.

CHAPTER 11

Hypertension

An elevated blood pressure is a frequent and significant finding that requires thoughtful and careful elucidation. It has important implications with regard to both cause and effect, with the consequences often being of more concern than the specific etiology.

Soon after completing your initial instruction in clinical diagnosis you are asked to perform a routine physical examination on an apparently healthy 40-year-old man who had volunteered his services for this purpose.

You find his blood pressure to be 160/110 mm Hg in his right arm when he is supine.

DIAGNOSTIC AND PROGNOSTIC FACTORS IN HYPERTENSION

Is this normal?

Epidemiologic studies in various communities have established a range of "normal" blood pressures for different age groups. The upper limit of normal in the adult has been *arbitrarily* set at 140/90 mm Hg, so that the simplistic answer is *yes*. A blood pressure reading of 160/110 mm Hg is abnormal.

How should you proceed?

- It is important to confirm the accuracy of the observation, and to exclude the possibility of artifact.

- If it proves to be a genuine finding, you must decide whether it is clinically significant and hence worthy of further pursuit.

Under what circumstances might an elevation of the blood pressure be artifactual?

- The instrument may be faulty.
- The cuff may be inappropriate to the patient—a standard-sized cuff applied to the large arm of an obese or muscular patient will result in a falsely high blood pressure reading.
- Your technique of blood pressure measurement may be imperfect. A falsely high pressure might result, for example:
  - From incorrect application of the cuff, if the cuff is too loose, or is not completely emptied of air.
  - Following repeated blood pressure determinations without removing and reapplying the cuff.
  - From incorrect positioning of the patient. In a recumbent patient, the blood pressure reading would be falsely high if the arm were held vertically downward.

Is this observation clinically significant?

- The level of the blood pressure reading per se is an important determining factor in this regard. The higher the pressure, the more clear-cut is its significance. A reading of 240/140 mm Hg should sound alarm bells in your mind. A pressure of 160/110 mm Hg is certainly significant.
- Since normal blood pressure increases with age, age is another important determining factor. A pressure reading of 150/95 mm Hg in a man of 80 would be of little concern, while the same level in a child (or in a pregnant female) would be important.
- The effects of hypertension in a male are perhaps more severe, so his sex contributes to the significance of the finding.
- A persistent elevation of the blood pressure is probably more important than a transient rise. If this abnormally high reading of 160/110 were to be confirmed later in the examination and/or on subsequent examinations, it would be more apt to be significant than would a single abnormal recording, with subsequent normal values.

- Evidence of "hypertensive disease", *i.e.,* complications of hypertension, renders a high blood pressure reading clinically significant, so that once high blood pressure has been noted, the history and physical examination *must* be geared toward seeking such evidence.

Why is the detection of hypertension important?

Insurance company statistics demonstrate that hypertension reduces life expectancy. By having detected hypertension in this asymptomatic patient, you may be in a position to improve his prognosis by reducing the risk of vascular complications.

However, not every hypertensive subject requires therapy, and you might do harm by alarming him unnecessarily, or by treating him inappropriately, or, in fact, at all.

Thus, having made the observation (and more particularly so if you were his primary physician), you are faced with the decision of what to tell the patient, and how to treat him. This requires knowledge of prognostic factors, and information on current management programs of hypertension, and their advantages and disadvantages.

Sustained high blood pressure, *irrespective of its cause,* is liable to be complicated by the development of secondary disease in a variety of organs and body systems.

Having detected an elevation in the blood pressure, it therefore behooves you, very consciously and specifically, to determine whether such complications exist. Their presence significantly influences the prognosis with regard to hypertension. They can themselves prove incapacitating and even fatal, and if present would constitute separate problems, each requiring a decision as to further investigation and management.

Much of the treatment of hypertension is aimed at preventing the development of such complications or, if already present, reversing them, or reducing their rate of progress. A component of the long-term management of a hypertensive patient is the early detection of the development, or progression, of such complications. In this context, careful initial and interval evaluation of a hypertensive patient is obviously important.

Hypertension may constitute a clue to a significant underlying disease process. In certain instances, cure or control of this process may be possible, sometimes with control of the hypertension also.

Thus, despite the fact that your "patient" is apparently well and asymptomatic, and that the abnormal finding was detected during a routine physical examination, hypertension should very realistically be formulated as a problem demanding further evaluation. This requires that you assess the patient as to

- The presence and extent of the *effects* of hypertension, and
- Its possible *causes*

To do so requires

- That you *know* what these causes and effects are
- That you *know*, and *can recognize* their clinical (and laboratory) manifestations, and
- That you employ a reasonable, systematic, and reliable system in order to detect them

EFFECTS OF HYPERTENSION

What are the potential effects of hypertension?

- The development of "hypertensive disease," including
  - Heart disease
  - Cerebrovascular disease
  - Retinal abnormalities
  - Renal disease
- The exacerbation of atherosclerotic vascular disease, manifesting clinically, particularly as
  - Ischemic heart disease
  - Cerebrovascular disease, and
  - Peripheral vascular disease

What are the clinical features of hypertensive heart disease?

Work hypertrophy of the left ventricle, which may in turn be complicated by

- Left heart failure, and then
- Right heart failure

What are the clinical features of hypertensive cerebrovascular disease?

- Headache

- Transient ischemic attacks
- Completed strokes
- Hypertensive encephalopathy

What are the retinal changes resulting from hypertension?

- Changes in the light reflex of vessels
- Arteriovenous nicking
- Hemorrhages and exudates
- Papilledema

These signs reflect the severity of the hypertensive process in a graduated fashion.

What are the features of hypertensive renal disease?

- Renal insufficiency
- Proteinuria
- An abnormal urinary sediment

It is eminently reasonable that you interview and examine your patient (and if necessary, reinterview and reexamine him), looking very specifically for those symptoms and signs that will allow you to detect and assess the presence and extent of the complications of hypertension.

How might you reasonably structure the interview in this regard?

Essentially, by utilizing a thoughtful and *selective* **REVIEW OF SYSTEMS** and **PAST HISTORY.** A review of symptoms relevant to the CARDIOVASCULAR SYSTEM might reveal the presence of

- Hypertensive heart disease
- Ischemic heart disease, and
- Occlusive peripheral vascular disease

A review of symptoms relevant to the CENTRAL NERVOUS SYSTEM might reveal the presence of

- Cerebrovascular complications

**From a consideration of symptoms relevant to the CARDIOVAS-
CULAR SYSTEM, what symptoms will suggest:**

1. **Left Heart Failure?**

   - A progressive ease of fatigability and effort dyspnea—with
     ultimately dyspnea even at rest
   - Orthopnea
   - Paroxysmal nocturnal dyspnea
   - Episodes of pulmonary edema

2. **Right Heart Failure?**

   - Dyspnea on effort
   - Ankle edema

3. **Ischemic Heart Disease?**

   - Angina pectoris
   - Palpitations, and a **PAST HISTORY** of myocardial in-
     farction

4. **Occlusive Peripheral Vascular Disease?**

   - Intermittent claudication
   - Coldness or numbness of the feet
   - Trophic changes and color changes in the feet, and a **PAST
     HISTORY** of gangrene, or of an amputation

**From a consideration of symptoms relevant to the CENTRAL
NERVOUS SYSTEM, what symptoms would suggest:**

1. **Hypertensive Headaches?**

   - A characteristic throbbing occipital headache present on
     awakening, and diminishing over the course of the day

2. **Transient Ischemic Attacks?**

   - Transient episodes of loss of function, or impaired function,
     of those areas of the brain where the blood supply is com-
     promised manifest by varying combinations of

     ○ Dysphasia
     ○ Visual disturbances
     ○ Hearing disturbances and tinnitus

  ○ Vertigo and disturbances of balance
  ○ Dysarthria
  ○ Parasthesias of the face and/or extremities
  ○ Weakness of the face and/or extremities

3. A Completed Stroke?

  • Persistence of the symptoms noted above, and more particu-
    larly, a mono- or hemi-paresis, and a **PAST HISTORY** of a
    stroke, or strokes.

4. Hypertensive Encephalopathy?

  • This is a very unlikely event to emerge from routine ques-
    tioning in a "healthy" subject with only moderate hyper-
    tension, and would be of far more concern in an ill subject
    with severe hypertension.

Symptoms that should alert you to this possibility would include:

  • Severe headache
  • Visual problems, and
  • Complaints of focal and transient cerebral dysfunction

—as above.

In addition:

  • Gastrointestinal symptoms—nausea and vomiting—might
    be present.

What symptoms would suggest renal dysfunction?

This is unlikely to be prominent, but review of symptoms
relevant to the GENITOURINARY SYSTEM might reveal

  • Nocturia
  • Polyuria, and
  • Frequency of micturition

Exceptionally, oliguria, anuria, or hematuria may occur as
manifestations of serious renal complications of hypertension
and atherosclerosis.

How might you reasonably structure the physical examination?

The usual systematic physical examination is admirably suited to this purpose, with particular attention being directed to the presence of specific signs.

These signs and their potential significance in the context of the patient with hypertension are shown in Table 11-1.

TABLE 11-1. PHYSICAL SIGNS OF POTENTIAL CLINICAL SIGNIFICANCE WHEN ATTEMPTING TO ASSESS THE EFFECTS OF HYPERTENSION

Source	Sign	Potential significance
General appearance	Head of bed elevated	Orthopnea and left heart failure
Mental status	Abnormal mental status, drowsiness, stupor or coma	Cerebrovascular accident Hypertensive encephalopathy
Vital signs		
PULSE	Tachycardia Pulsus alternans	Heart failure
Head		
EYE	Hypertensive retinopathy	Important implications concerning the severity of the process
	Nystagmus	Cerebrovascular disease
FACE	Cranial nerve palsies	Cerebrovascular disease
NECK	Jugular venous pressure elevation	Right heart failure
	Carotid bruits	Atherosclerotic disease
Precordium		
INSPECTION AND PALPA- TION	Prominence and lateral displacement of the apex beat	Left ventricular strain and hypertrophy
AUSCULTA- TION	Prominance of A2	High aortic pressure
	An S4 gallop	Diminished left ventricular disten- sibility
	Early diastolic aortic murmur	Aortic root dilatation
	An S3 gallop	Ventricular failure
	A systolic murmur	Mitral ring dilatation resulting from ventricular failure and dilatation
Lung fields	Basal crackles	Left heart failure
	Signs of pleural effusion	Right heart failure
Abdomen	Hepatomegaly Ascites	Right heart failure

(continued)

TABLE 11-1. PHYSICAL SIGNS OF POTENTIAL CLINICAL
SIGNIFICANCE WHEN ATTEMPTING TO ASSESS THE EFFECTS
OF HYPERTENSION *(Continued)*

Source	Sign	Potential significance
Extremities **Circulatory** **system**		

INSPECTION	Pallor of the skin
	Discoloration of the skin
	Trophic changes—
	  including ulceration
	  and gangrene
		Occlusive peripheral
		vascular disease

PALPATION	Coldness of a limb Absent or diminished pulses	
AUSCULTA- TION	Femoral artery bruits	
INSPECTION AND PALPA- TION	Edema	Heart failure

Nervous
system
	Sensory loss
	Ataxia
	Upper motor neuron
	  pathology:
	    Weakness
	    "Increased tone"
	    Hyper-reflexia
	    Abnormal reflexes
		Cerebrovascular disease

Which laboratory studies might contribute to the initial assessment of the effects of hypertension?

- Urinalysis
- Serum creatinine and BUN assays
- Chest radiograph
- Electrocardiogram

CAUSES OF HYPERTENSION

Having considered the effects of hypertension, you now need to consider its possible causes in relation to your patient.

What is the most common cause?

- Idiopathic hypertension

What other causes are important, particularly because they may be correctable?

- Renal disease—especially if unilateral
- Coarctation of the aorta
- Endocrine disorders
  - Cushing's syndrome
  - Pheochromocytoma
  - Aldosteronism
- Drug or food use
  - Oral contraceptives
  - Steroids
  - Licorice
  - Monoamine oxidase (MAO) inhibitors

How might the HISTORY be constructed and utilized to help determine which of these causes is operative?

A consideration of the **PROBLEM LIST** (or **PAST HISTORY**) might reveal prior documentation of a disorder or circumstances known to be associated with hypertension, *e.g.*:

- Previous renal disease, or renovascular trauma
- A psychiatric disorder likely to be treated with MAO inhibitors

A **REVIEW OF SYSTEMS** might reveal, with regard to

1. The General Health

- Episodic palpitations or fatigue, and/or
- Weight loss, and/or
- Sweating

—all suggestive of a pheochromocytoma.

- Episodic muscular weakness, suggestive of aldosteronism
- Weakness and fatigue, suggestive of Cushing's syndrome

2. The Genitourinary System

- Flank pain
- Ureteral colic
- Suprapubic discomfort or pain

- Hematuria
- Frequency
- Polyuria
- Nocturia and dysuria

—all suggestive of possible urinary tract disease. (Polyuria and nocturia, possibly consequent on hypokalemia, would also suggest aldosteronism or Cushing's syndrome.)

- Impotence (and amenorrhea, in a female)—suggestive of Cushing's syndrome

These various symptoms could, however, equally reflect the *consequences* of hypertension, and have no bearing on cause.

The **DRUG** and **FOOD HISTORY** might reveal

- Oral contraceptive use
- Use of MAO inhibitors
- Ingestion of licorice
- Steroid administration

All of these might be causative.

THE FAMILY HISTORY might reveal

- A history of hypertension, strokes, and heart disease in other members of the family, which would support a diagnosis of essential hypertension.
- A diagnosis of a pheochromocytoma in other family members, which would render pheochromocytoma a strong diagnostic possibility.

How might you reasonably structure the physical examination when trying to determine the cause of the hypertension?

Again, the systematic physical examination is suited to this purpose, with particular attention being directed toward detecting specific signs.

These signs and their potential significance are shown in the Table 11-2.

Are any laboratory studies indicated in this initial assessment of etiology?

- Assay of the serum potassium creatinine and BUN concentrations

TABLE 11-2. SIGNS OF POTENTIAL DIAGNOSTIC SIGNIFICANCE
IN THE PATIENT WITH HYPERTENSION

Source	Sign	Potential significance
General appearance	Truncal obesity Weight loss	Cushing's syndrome Pheochromocytoma
Vital signs	Fever Tachycardia	Pheochromocytoma
Head and neck	"Moon" facies Acneiform rash Plethoric facies "Buffalo" hump	Cushing's syndrome
Thorax	Intercostal pulsations	Coarctation of the aorta
Abdomen	Purple striae Palpable kidney Arterial bruits	Cushing's syndrome Renal disease
Extremities	Radiofemoral arterial pulse delay Diminished or absent femoral pulses	Coarctation of the aorta

- Urinalysis, including culture
- Radiograph of abdomen for kidney size estimate

If no positive information were forthcoming, this might well
serve as the total evaluation of the patient with regard to a
possible cause for his hypertension.

Conversely, if, for example, he admitted to episodic palpitations
and flushing, and/or had lost weight, and/or had a brother with a
pheochromocytoma, this would obviously require that you very
seriously consider the possibility of his having a pheochromocytoma, and that you structure your further investigation around
this possibility—reading about it, asking about it, learning about
the investigations, their risks, their reliability, their cost, the
subsequent management of the patient, etc.

You should now be in the position to know:

- The nature (if any), and the extent, of the complications of
  hypertension in this patient—and hence have some idea as to
  prognosis and treatment;
- Whether there is a need for further investigation of the
  etiology.

CHAPTER 12

Hypotension

A sudden fall in blood pressure usually constitutes a critical situation that demands urgent diagnosis and treatment. Sometimes the cause and its treatment are obvious. In other circumstances they may be far from clear.

Immediate transfer to a critical care facility, with the application of sophisticated monitoring equipment, is often required.

While an intern in the hematology-oncology department, you are called to the emergency room to see a 43-year-old woman with breast cancer, well known to the department, who has had several episodes of syncope over the past 3 days, and whose blood pressure is 90/40 mm Hg. Previous blood pressure recordings in the chart range between 120/75 and 140/80 mm Hg.

CAUSES OF HYPOTENSION

What basic mechanisms to account for the patient's hypotension might you reasonably consider, on your way to the emergency room?

It is useful to consider a model of the circulatory system. In Figure 12-1, the circulatory system is compared to a mechanical pumping system, and the potential for problems at a variety of sites is shown:

- The pump may be at fault—secondary to either an electrical or a mechanical problem.
- There may be an obstruction to flow, either into, or out of, the pump.

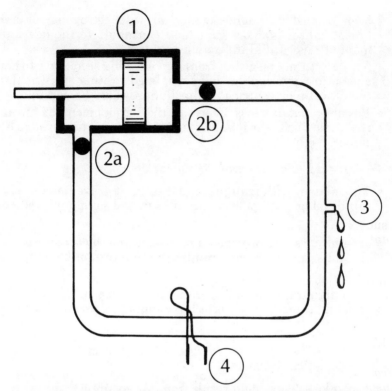

FIG. 12-1. Schematic representation of the heart and circulation, useful to the evaluation of hypotension. (*1*) Pump defect; (*2a*) obstruction to flow *into* the heart (pump); (*2b*) obstruction to flow *out of* the heart (pump); (*3*) loss of blood volume; (*4*) diminished peripheral resistance.

- The circulating fluid may be diminished in volume.
- The resistance to flow may be diminished.

In view of the diagnosis of breast cancer in this patient, what causes for *her* being hypotensive would you consider?

With regard to pump failure:

- *Myocardial infarction* is a common disease and should always be considered in a hypotensive subject. In this patient the risk is perhaps slightly increased, since she may have been treated by oophorectomy, *or* with estrogens for her breast cancer—factors that may contribute to the development of myocardial infarction in a female.

- An arrhythmia resulting from hypokalemia secondary to her chemotherapy should be considered. Either ventricular tachycardia or ventricular fibrillation would be possible.
- Possible, but far less likely, is the devèlopment of an arrhythmia due to the involvement of the conducting system by tumor.

With regard to obstruction to blood flow:

- This patient with malignant disease is at grave risk for having developed deep vein thrombosis and pulmonary embolism.

- Inferior or superior vena caval obstruction by tumor and/or thrombus might have diminished the return of blood to the heart.

- A malignant, or a radiation-induced pericarditis, with effusion and tamponade, might have compromised cardiac function

With regard to a reduction in fluid volume, the patient may have volume depletion, because of

- Blood loss. This could result from, for example:
  ○ Steroid, analgesic, or stress-related peptic ulceration
  ○ Disease, or treatment-related thrombocytopenia
  ○ Disseminated intravascular coagulation
  ○ Bleeding from tumor sites
- Fluid loss. This could result from
  ○ Anorexia, nausea, vomiting, and diarrhea—due to a variety of possible factors (see Chapter 6).
- Adrenal dysfunction—perhaps resulting from surgical adrenalactomy, treatment with aminoglutethimide, or involvement of the adrenal glands by tumor.

With regard to a reduction in peripheral resistance:

- She is especially at risk for gram-negative septicemia, because
  ○ Chemotherapy and/or radiotherapy, or
  ○ Marrow infiltration by tumor

—might each be responsible for significant neutropenia, which is eminently liable to complication by sepsis.

- Her medication might be responsible for autonomic dysfunction—hence a reduction in peripheral resistance:
  - ○ Vincristine might well comprise part of her treatment regime, and this drug is known to be responsible for postural hypotension.
  - ○ Sedative or tranquillizing drugs, or antidepressant drugs might have been prescribed, and her hypotension could be a side effect of their action.
  - ○ An anaphylactic response should always be considered.
- Hypoadrenalism may operate in part through this mechanism to lower the blood pressure.

When you arrive in the emergency room and see the patient, how should you proceed?

- First you should assess the urgency of the situation.
- Her blood pressure and state of consciousness should be checked.
- Simple postural treatment—elevating the foot of the bed—if not already effected, should be instituted.
- An intravenous line should be established.
- Admission to an intensive care facility for monitoring purposes should be considered.
- A diagnosis should be established as quickly as possible, from a consideration of the main diagnostic possibilities of
  - ○ Blood loss
  - ○ Pulmonary embolism
  - ○ Septicemia
  - ○ Myocardial infarction

and remembering also

- ○ Fluid loss
- ○ Hypoadrenalism
- ○ Peripheral vasodilatation
- ○ Pericardial tamponade
- ○ A significant arrhythmia

How might the HISTORY help to differentiate among these conditions?

The **REVIEW OF SYSTEMS** might reveal, with regard to

1. Her General Health

- Fever—suggestive of an infection, and hence septicemia; and perhaps of pulmonary embolism

2. The Gastrointestinal Tract

- Hematemesis,
- Melena, or
- Passage of fresh blood per rectum

all obviously indicative of blood loss.

- Anorexia, with diminished fluid intake
- Vomiting, or
- Diarrhea

—suggestive of a depleted fluid volume.

- Dyspepsia—possibly suggestive of blood loss from as yet occult gastrointestinal bleeding.

3. The Cardiovascular System

- Central chest pain—suggestive of myocardial infarction, pulmonary embolism, and possibly pericarditis
- Pain and/or swelling in a lower limb—very suggestive of pulmonary embolism following deep vein thrombosis

4. The Respiratory System

Recent sudden, episodic, or progressive

- Dyspnea—suggestive of pulmonary embolism or myocardial infarction; and possibly of pneumonia, and hence of septicemia
- Pleuritic chest pain
- Wheezing
- Cough, and/or
- Hemoptysis

—all suggestive of pulmonary embolism; and pneumonia and septicemia.

A review of the **DRUG HISTORY** might reveal

- Recent chemotherapeutic drug administration (or radiotherapy), with its consequent risks of
  - Neutropenia, and hence septicemia
  - Thrombocytopenia, and hence blood loss
  - Peptic ulceration—and blood loss
  - Peripheral vasodilatation
  - Radiation-induced pericarditis and tamponade
- Sedative, antidepressant, analgesic, or antiemetic drug ingestion—with their consequent risks of
  - Peptic ulceration—and blood loss
  - Peripheral vasodilatation
- Use of aminoglutethimide, or a surgical adrenalectomy—with the attendant potential consequences of hypoadrenalism
- Use of diuretics, or other antihypertensive medication—with the possible effects of fluid depletion or peripheral vasodilatation

How might the PHYSICAL EXAMINATION contribute to the diagnosis?

It might reveal, with regard to

1. Her Vital Signs

- A pyrexia—suggestive of infection; or embolism
- A pulse
  - With a bounding character, and associated with a warm, dry periphery, indicative of peripheral vasodilatation, hence probable sepsis, or a possible drug effect
  - Small and thready, associated with a cold, clammy periphery, hence suggestive of blood loss, or fluid depletion, infarct, or pulmonary embolism
  - Paradoxical—suggestive of pericardial tamponade
  - Significantly fast; slow; or irregular
- Tachypnea—compatible with pulmonary embolism, pneumonia, myocardial infarction, or significant blood loss
- Confirmation (or detection) of a paradoxical pulse on measuring the blood pressure—and also suggestive of tamponade

2. Her Head and Neck

- Pallor—suggestive of blood loss, but also compatible with compensatory vasoconstriction
- Loss of eyeball tension—indicative of severe dehydration
- A dry mouth—also suggestive of dehydration, but compatible with tachypnea or hyperpnea
- Significant elevation of the jugular venous pressure, with the presence of Kussmaul's sign and a rapid "y" descent, suggestive of tamponade; or
- A large "a" wave, suggestive of pulmonary embolism.

3. Her Thorax

- The presence of a pleural friction rub—very suggestive of pulmonary embolism in this patient with hypotension. (It could equally reflect a malignant pleural effusion and have no bearing on the immediate problem.)
- Basal crepitations—possibly suggestive of myocardial infarction
- Signs of consolidation—suggestive of pneumonia, hence septicemia; also of pulmonary embolism

4. Her Precordium

- An "absent" apex beat
- An increased area of cardiac dullness to percussion,
- A muffled intensity of the heart sounds, and/or
- A pericardial friction rub

—all very suggestive of malignant pericarditis and tamponade.

- A gallop rhythm—suggestive of pulmonary embolism or myocardial infarction
- An arrhythmia—which may be more easily discernible on auscultation of the heart than by palpation of the pulse, and which may complicate myocardial infarction or pulmonary embolism, or reflect the effects of hypokalemia or malignant disease of the conducting system.
- A right ventricular lift to the left of the sternum, a palpable P2, a loud P2, a right atrial gallop, or pulmonary murmurs—suggestive of pulmonary embolism

5. Her Abdomen

- Abdominal distention—suggestive of possible intraperitoneal blood loss or vincristine-associated ileus

- Hepatomegaly—perhaps suggestive of tamponade but quite probably resulting from metastatic disease. A pulsatile enlargement of the liver might suggest acute cor pulmonale due to embolism, with dilation of the tricuspid ring.
- Increased bowel sounds—suggestive of gastrointestinal bleeding

6. The Rectal Examination

- Evidence of melena or fresh blood—obviously very suggestive of gastrointestinal bleeding

7. The Extremities

- A Swollen and/or tender lower limb—very suggestive of deep vein thrombosis, hence of pulmonary embolism

8. The Skin

- Loss of skin turgor—suggestive of dehydration, but possibly resulting from tissue wasting associated with the malignant process
- Evidence of a bleeding tendency—bruises, hematomas, a petechial rash, oozing from venipuncture sites—suggestive of blood loss as the cause of the hypotension; but also of septicemia—and the associated disseminated intravascular coagulation

What initial laboratory studies are indicated?

- A full blood count
- An electrocardiogram
- A chest radiograph

On further evaluation of your patient you learn that she has been febrile for 2 days. Her last course of chemotherapy, comprising cyclophosphamide, 5-fluorouracil and methotrexate, had been administered 10 days previously. She has recently developed a nonproductive cough. Her left leg has been painful for 3 days. She is tachypneic. Her leukocyte count is 800/cu mm.

What is the differential diagnosis, in light of this information?

Septicemia must be considered, in view of the fever and significant neutropenia. The cough suggests pneumonia as the possible source.

Pulmonary embolism should also be considered. The cough, the tachypnea, and the painful leg must alert you to this possibility in a hypotensive subject.

How should you proceed?

- To a history and physical examination, looking for confirmatory evidence of septicemia, and its probable pneumonic basis
- To a physical examination, looking for confirmatory evidence of pulmonary embolism
- To laboratory data in support of these two diagnostic possibilities

What signs, in addition to fever and hypotension, would support a diagnosis of septicemia?

With regard to the

- Pulse
  - Tachycardia
  - A full, bounding quality
- Skin
  - A warm, dry periphery
  - A pustular rash
  - Ecthyma gangrenosum
  - Bruising, and/or oozing from venipuncture sites
  - A petechial rash

What additional signs would support a diagnosis of pulmonary embolism?

See Chapter 5.

What further laboratory investigations are indicated in this patient?

- Blood cultures
- Repeat chest radiographs

- A lung scan
- Blood gas determinations
- A coagulation profile seeking evidence of disseminated intravascular coagulation

Why is a correct diagnosis important?

It is essential to the rapid institution of appropriate therapy. Therapy is urgently indicated, and is usually beneficial. Inappropriate therapy can be catastrophic.

EFFECTS OF HYPOTENSION

What are the potential consequences of such hypertension?

- Impaired consciousness
- Renal failure
- Impaired lung function
- Liver failure
- Myocardial infarction
- Complications of therapy
- Death

How may these be assessed?

By the following, if necessary:

- Repeated mental status examination
- Careful monitoring of the fluid intake and output; and serial BUN and creatinine determinations
- Serial blood gas determinations
- Frequent examination for evidence of asterixis, abnormal mental function, jaundice, and fetor hepaticus
- Examination for symptoms and signs of myocardial infarction, and repeated electrocardiograms
- Careful monitoring of

○ Central venous pressure
○ Pulmonary wedge pressures
○ Heart rate and rhythm
○ Blood pressure
○ Blood counts
○ Electrolytes
- By being aware of, and looking for, the potential side effects of the therapeutic agents and maneuvers that you are employing

CHAPTER 13

Clubbing of the Fingers

Clubbing is an important physical sign. The routine physical examination should include a search for its presence.

If detected, it always demands an investigation as to its underlying cause. Such investigation logically begins with the history and physical examination, highlighting those aspects relevant to the probable causes.

During a clinical diagnosis exercise you see a 45-year-old man who is in the hospital "for investigation." Your instructor suggests that you first examine his hands, and that you base the remainder of the interview and examination on the findings you elicit.

You notice definite "clubbing" of the patient's fingers.

What is the clinical significance of "clubbing"?

While innocuous in itself, and while the patient is usually unaware of the phenomenon, clubbing almost always implies significant underlying pathology.

What are its probable causes?

Clubbing may be caused by diseases of the lungs and pleura, diseases of the heart, and by certain other disease conditions. More specifically, these conditions include:

1. Diseases of the Lungs and Pleura

- Malignant disease

- ○ Usually bronchogenic carcinoma
- ○ Occasionally, lymphoma
- ● "Purulent" disease
  - ○ Lung abscess
  - ○ Empyema
  - ○ Bronchiectasis
- ● Other lung diseases
  - ○ Some pneumoconioses
  - ○ Some infiltrating processes, but
  - ○ *Not* chronic obstructive pulmonary disease per se

2. Diseases of the Heart
- ● Congenital cyanotic heart disease
- ● Bacterial endocarditis

3. Other Disorders
- ● Primary biliary cirrhosis
- ● Chronic inflammatory bowel disease
- ● A familial tendency toward finger clubbing
- ● Certain rare disease conditions

How might the HISTORY help in differentiating between these various disorders?

The **SYSTEMS REVIEW** might reveal, with regard to

1. His General Health
- ● Fever
- ● Malaise
- ● Fatigue
- ● Weight loss
- ● Anorexia

—suggestive of infection or malignant disease.

2. The Cardiovascular System
- ● Chest pain
- ● Dyspnea
- ● Palpitations
- ● Edema

- Squatting

—suggestive of heart disease.

3. The Respiratory System

- Dyspnea
- Cough
- Sputum production
- Hemoptysis
- Chest pain
- Wheezing, or
- Hoarseness

—all suggestive of disease of the lungs or pleura.

If the sputum were purulent (and even more so if it were putrid), this would increase the likelihood of a lung abscess, or bronchiectasis. Hemopytsis would suggest both bronchiectasis and a bronchogenic carcinoma, and perhaps a lung abscess.

4. The Gastrointestinal System

- Jaundice—suggestive of primary biliary cirrhosis, but also of metastatic involvement of the liver by lung tumor, or possibly lymphoma
- Diarrhea—especially if associated with the passage of blood and mucus—suggestive of chronic inflammatory bowel disease

5. The Skin and Musculoskeletal Systems

- Pruritus, or bone pain—symptoms suggestive of primary biliary cirrhosis, or metastatic lung cancer
- Arthralgia—perhaps suggestive of chronic inflammatory bowel disease, or endocarditis

6. The Genitourinary System

- Hematuria—suggestive of endocarditis

The **PAST HISTORY**, or **REVIEW OF THE PROBLEM LIST** might reveal a history of

- Known lung or heart disease, or
- Previous lung or heart surgery

—circumstances that would strongly incriminate disease of one or other of these organs as the source of the clubbing.

- Previous rheumatic fever—rendering bacterial endocarditis an eminently likely cause
- Previous measles, whooping cough, or tuberculosis—which would increase the possibility of bronchiectasis
- Recurrent sinusitis—also suggestive of associated bronchiectasis
- Recurrent bouts of pneumonia, especially if the same anatomical site were involved—which would be very suggestive of both bronchiectasis and bronchogenic carcinoma
- Recent loss of consciousness, anesthesia, vomiting, or choking—all likely to be complicated by aspiration and the subsequent development of a lung abscess
- Recent dental work (or lack thereof)—which might be complicated both by aspiration and a lung abscess, and by the development of bacterial endocarditis

The **FAMILY HISTORY** might reveal documentation in other family members of

- Cystic fibrosis, or
- Agammaglobulinemia

—hence suggesting their possible presence, with complicating bronchiectasis, in your patient.

Review of the **LIFE SITUATION** might reveal evidence of **OCCUPATIONAL** exposure to

- Asbestos—suggestive of lung cancer, or
- Other dusts—suggestive of a pneumoconiosis

Review of the patient's **HABITS** might reveal

- Alcohol excesses—suggestive of a possible lung abscess
- Cigarette smoking—suggestive of lung cancer; and/or
- Drug addiction, especially "mainlining,"—which would render bacterial endocarditis very probable

Upon interviewing your patient, you learn that he had rheumatic fever at the age of ten. There were no apparent aftereffects. Three months ago he had some dental work done under local anesthetic. Since that time he has been a "little under the weather," and perhaps feverish and sweaty at times. He has lost 6-7 lbs.

What diagnosis does this history suggest?

- Subacute bacterial endocarditis!
- (A lung abscess following the dental work is a more remote possibility.)

What signs will you look for specifically, in the PHYSICAL EXAMINA-TION, to support this diagnostic hypothesis?

With regard to his

1. **Vital Signs**

   - Pyrexia
   - Pulse
     - Tachycardia
     - Abnormalities suggestive of valvular heart disease: *e.g.*, a collapsing pulse

2. **Hand**

   - Splinter hemorrhages in the fingernails
   - Osler's nodes
   - Janeway's spots

3. **Skin**

   - Petechiae

4. **Head and Neck**

   - Petechial hemorrhages—characteristically involving the conjunctival mucous membranes, also the buccal mucosa
   - Fundal hemorrhages (Roth spots)
   - Pallor of the mucous membranes
   - Abnormalities of the jugular venous pressure and pulse, indicative of underlying valvular heart disease
   - Focal neurologic signs (resulting from emboli)

5. **Precordium**

   - Abnormalities of the apex beat
   - Abnormalities of the heart sounds—especially the presence of cardiac murmurs

6. Abdomen

- Splenomegaly

7. Extremities

- Focal neurologic signs resulting from embolism

If these supportive signs are evident—and even if they are not—what laboratory studies are indicated?

- A complete blood count
- Urinalysis—looking for both hematuria and other features of acute diffuse glomerulonephritis
- Repeated blood cultures
- A chest radiograph

Had the history failed to reveal significant leads, what features in the PHYSICAL EXAMINATION might you assess for diagnostic clues?

With regard to

1. His General Appearance and Environment

- An appearance of "chronic ill health" might indicate infection or malignancy.
- A foul odor in the room would suggest a lung abscess.
- Inspection of the *sputum* cup might reveal
  - Purulent sputum, suggestive of bronchiectasis or a lung abscess; or
  - Blood, suggestive of malignancy or bronchiectasis

2. His Vital Signs

- Fever would be suggestive of
  - Lung abscess
  - Bronchiectasis
  - Empyema
  - Endocarditis
  - Lung cancer/lymphoma

3. His Hands

- Splinter hemorrhages, Osler's nodes, and Janeway's spots would be suggestive of endocarditis.

- Palmar xanthomata would be very suggestive of primary biliary cirrhosis.

4. His Head and Neck

- Jaundice would be suggestive of biliary cirrhosis.
- Signs of endocarditis might be evident (see above).
- A Horner's syndrome would be highly suggestive of lung cancer, or a lymphoma.
- Cyanosis would be strongly suggestive of congenital cyanotic heart disease, and possibly of pulmonary disease.
- Dental caries and periodontal disease would suggest a lung abscess.
- Cervical adenopathy would be very suggestive of a bronchogenic carcinoma, or of a lymphoma.

5. His Lung Fields

- Asymmetry
- Abnormalities of
  - Respiratory excursion
  - The percussion note
  - The intensity of the breath sounds
  - Vocal resonance or fremitus
- Adventitious sounds

—would indicate diseases of the lungs or pleura.

6. His Precordium

- Displacement or abnormal character of the apex beat would suggest
  - Heart disease, or lung cancer complicated by atelectasis or a pleural effusion
- Abnormal heart sounds, or cardiac murmurs, would indicate heart disease.
- Dextrocardia would suggest bronchiectasis (Kartagener's syndrome).

7. His Abdomen

- Hepatomegaly might be associated with primary biliary cirrhosis, metastatic lung cancer, or lymphoma.
- Splenomegaly might indicate endocarditis or primary biliary cirrhosis.

- Masses or tenderness to palpation might suggest chronic inflammatory bowel disease.

8. The Rectal Examination

- The presence of
  - ○ Fissures
  - ○ Ulcers
  - ○ Fistulae
  - ○ Blood and mucus in the stool

—would all suggest chronic inflammatory bowel disease.

While examining the patient's chest, you detect dullness to percussion over the right lower chest.

In the context of this patient with clubbing of the fingers, what is the potential significance of this finding?

It may reflect:

- An empyema
- Pneumonic consolidation complicating bronchiectasis
- A lung abscess
- A variety of possible complications of lung cancer
  - ○ A pleural effusion
  - ○ Pulmonary atelectasis
  - ○ Pneumonic consolidation
  - ○ Pulmonary fibrosis in a localized region
  - ○ A malignant pericardial effusion
  - ○ Phrenic nerve paralysis with elevation of the hemidiaphragm
  - ○ Elevation of the diaphragm by massive hepatomegaly

The logical next step is to try to differentiate between these various causes for dullness to percussion of the chest, which is the subject of the next chapter.

CHAPTER 14

Dullness to Percussion (of the Chest)

Dullness to percussion is a significant physical sign elicited during percussion of the chest over areas that normally produce resonant sounds. The change may be subtle, or quite obvious.

This sign is sometimes detected in the course of a routine physical examination, and may thus be the first clue to the existence of significant pathology.

Conversely, as in the patient described in the previous chapter, detection of this sign often helps to confirm a tentative diagnosis of chest pathology.

Whatever the circumstances of its detection, its cause must always be explained.

What disorders can account for this finding of dullness to percussion on examination of the chest?

Any circumstance that causes air-filled lung to be replaced by liquid or solid will manifest this sign. It is useful to consider potential causes along anatomic lines. Thus, there might be an abnormality of

- The underlying lung—resulting in
  - Pulmonary consolidation
  - Pulmonary fibrosis
- The airways—leading to
  - Atelectasis
- The pleura—with the development of
  - Pleural fluid

- ○ Pleural fibrosis and thickening
- • The phrenic nerve—causing paralysis and
  - ○ Elevation of the diaphragm
- • Subdiaphragmatic structures—with
  - ○ Splenomegaly
  - ○ Other masses
  - ○ Ascites
  - ○ Other causes for abdominal distention—resulting in eleva-
    tion of the diaphragm and compression of lung tissue

How might you attempt to decide which of these conditions is present?

- • Examination of the chest and abdomen usually will provide a specific answer.
- • Selected laboratory tests can be used to confirm the clinical diagnosis.

With regard to a careful examination of the chest, how might inspection contribute?

By revealing

- • Asymmetry of the chest contour, and/or
- • Diminished respiratory excursion on the ipsilateral side.

While neither of these signs serves a discriminatory function, each serves to support the contention of significant pulmonary or pleural pathology.

- • A mediastinal shift may be detected from displacement of the apex beat and trachea. This finding has great diagnostic importance.

Why is a shift of the apex beat or trachea of diagnostic significance?

It implies that the mediastinal structures have been either *pushed toward, or pulled away from,* one or other side of the chest—reflecting "space-occupying" pathology, or "loss" of tissue, respectively. (A shift in the position of the apex beat also could be a result of heart disease.)

What is the significance of a shift of the apex beat and trachea away from the area of dullness?

This would suggest the presence of

- Pleural fluid

(As an initial or isolated finding it would also suggest a pneumothorax, but in that circumstance, the percussion note would be hyperresonant and *not* dull.)

What is the significance of a shift *toward* the area of dullness?

This would suggest

- Atelectasis, or
- Localized pulmonary fibrosis

How may careful palpation help to elucidate the cause of the dullness to percussion?

Palpation should confirm the visual impression of diminished respiratory movement, or of displacement of the apex beat or trachea, or more readily reveal these changes.

Vocal fremitus may be altered over the area of dullness:

- Diminished fremitus would suggest
  - Pleural fluid
  - Pleural thickening
  - Elevation of the diaphragm, or
  - Atelectasis—if due to obstruction in the larger bronchi
- Increased fremitus would suggest
  - Consolidation
  - Atelectasis, with the larger bronchi patent
  - Localized pulmonary fibrosis

How might further percussion help?

If the area of the dullness were to change when the patient changes his position from sitting, to lying in the right or left lateral position, this would be very suggestive of a pleural effusion.

What might you learn from auscultation of the chest?

Changes in character of the breath sounds might occur.

- Their *intensity* might be diminished, suggesting
  - Pleural fluid
  - Pleural thickening
  - Elevation of the diaphragm, or
  - Atelectasis
- Their *quality* might be altered, with the production of *bronchial breathing,* suggesting
  - Consolidation
  - Atelectasis
  - Pulmonary fibrosis
  - Pleural fluid
  - A large pericardial effusion

Aside from changes in the breath sounds,

- *Additional sounds* might be audible in the form of a
  - *Pleural friction rub,* suggesting inflammatory disease of the pleura
  - *Crackles,* suggesting consolidation, atelectasis, or pulmonary fibrosis
- *Vocal resonance* might be decreased, or increased—with the same implications as altered vocal fremitus

What might be learned from examination of the abdomen?

- *Inspection* might reveal evidence of
  - Generalized abdominal distention, or
  - Asymmetry in the upper abdomen suggesting a mass in this region.
- *Palpation* might confirm (or reveal) the presence of a mass in the abdomen that might be responsible for an elevation of the diaphragm.
- *Percussion* might confirm or reveal the presence of ascites that could be responsible for elevation of the diaphragm.

What laboratory studies are indicated?

- A chest radiograph is essential.

A spectrum of "respiratory" findings might have been discovered through this examination. It would then be necessary to gear your thinking toward answering the question:

- Are the findings those of (for example)
  - Consolidation,
  - Pleural fluid, or
  - Atelectasis?

In order to answer this question, you must know the constellation of findings that reflect these conditions.

What are the findings of consolidation—

1. On inspection?

- Diminished respiratory movement of the ipsilateral chest
- Absence of mediastinal shift

2. On palpation?

- Confirmation of the above signs
- Increased vocal fremitus

3. On percussion?

- "Moderate" dullness

4. On auscultation?

- Bronchial breathing
- Crackles
- Increased vocal resonance
- Perhaps a pleural friction rub

What additional features might be contributory?

- A history of recent onset of fever, malaise, cough, chest pain
- Findings of fever, tachypnea, tachycardia, and flaring of the alae nasi
- Sputum production

What are the features of pleural fluid—

1. On inspection?

- Diminished unilateral respiratory excursion

- Sometimes a mediastinal shift away from that side. (With many effusions, however, this may not be evident.)

2. On palpation:

- Confirmation of the above signs
- Diminished vocal fremitus

3. On percussion?

- Stony dullness

4. On auscultation?

- Diminution in the intensity of the breath sounds
- Diminished vocal resonance
- Possibly an area of bronchial breathing, or crackles, *above* the level of the fluid
- Possibly a pleural friction rub

What are the features of *atelectasis* —

1. On inspection?

- Diminished unilateral respiratory excursion
- Mediastinal shift toward the pathology (sometimes)

2. On palpation?

- Confirmation of the above signs
- Usually diminished vocal fremitus, if the obstruction is in a major bronchus; possibly increased fremitus, if the obstruction is more distal

3. On percussion?

- Moderate dullness

4. On auscultation?

- Crackles
- Possibly bronchial breathing
- Possibly diminished intensity of breath sounds
- A variable change in vocal resonance

The chest radiograph will also contribute significantly to the differential diagnosis.

By this point you may have established that your patient has— for example—an accumulation of fluid in his pleural cavity that explains the dullness to percussion.

The next step will be to determine *its* cause.

CHAPTER 15

Pleural Fluid

Any of a number of initial clinical problems might ultimately be resolved by being ascribed to "pleural fluid." For example, "dyspnea on effort" or "dullness to percussion" might, with further information, be shown to result from fluid in the pleural cavity.

Once the presence of pleural fluid has been established, it then becomes necessary to determine *its* cause and effects.

What is the nature of the fluid that might accumulate in the pleural space?

- Blood—a hemothorax
- Chyle—a chylous effusion
- A transudate—a pleural effusion
- An exudate—a pleural effusion
- Pus—an empyema

How may these be differentiated?

- *From the clinical circumstances:*
  - A "pleural effusion" is by far the most common cause, and, in the absence of circumstances suggesting other conditions, will be the most likely.

Examples of circumstances suggesting other conditions include:

  - Recent trauma to the chest in the form of blunt injury, stab wounds, or surgery—a hemothorax would be more likely; a chylous effusion or an empyema would be possible.
  - Rupture of an aortic aneurysm, with its attendant pain and acute onset—a hemothorax would be probable.

○ A preceding staphylococcal pneumonia, particularly in a child, and especially if accompanied by a persistent "swinging" temperature, and the development of finger clubbing—an empyema would be probable.

○ Known malignant disease—malignant involvement of the lymphatic drainage of the chest might produce a chylous effusion.

Ultimate differentiation, if deemed necessary, will depend upon needle aspiration and analysis of the fluid.

What are the common and/or important causes of a pleural effusion?

The vast majority of effusions result from one of the following:

- Congestive heart failure
- Malignant disease
- Pneumonia
- Pulmonary embolism and infarction
- Trauma
- Tuberculosis
- Systemic lupus erythematosus

What other conditions may sometimes cause this condition?

Other causes to remember include:
- Subdiaphragmatic pathology
  ○ Subphrenic abscess
  ○ Amebic hepatitis
  ○ Pancreatitis
- Cirrhosis of the liver with ascites
- The nephrotic syndrome and other causes for hypoproteinemia
- Serum sickness and drug allergies

Are there other disorders that might be responsible?

Yes. Many! But these are much less frequent.

What are the major factors of value in the differential diagnosis of a pleural effusion?

These include:

- Age
- Sex
- Geography
- The associated clinical circumstances

How do these factors contribute?

1. Age

- In children and young adults:
  - ○ Preceding pneumonia would be most likely.
  - ○ Trauma would be a real possibility.
- In older age groups:
  - ○ Congestive heart failure, and
  - ○ Malignant disease

assume increasing importance.

2. Sex

- In young women, systemic lupus erythematosus should be considered.

3. Geography

- Immigration from, or recent travel to, areas where tuberculosis is endemic make tuberculosis a very real consideration. Similarly, amebic hepatitis, or coccidioidomycosis, might be likely in some patients under appropriate circumstances.

4. Associated Clinical Circumstances

- The clinical features associated with the development, or detection, of an effusion will usually be of great diagnostic significance, as shown in Table 15-1.

The following patient problem serves to illustrate the application of these principles:

A 42-year-old male singing teacher was perfectly well until 4 weeks prior to admission, when he began to develop increasing dyspnea on effort. He was referred to the Respiratory Outpatient Clinic, where physical examination and chest radiograph showed the features of a large amount of fluid in the right pleural cavity. He was admitted to the ward for further evaluation. As the intern in the department, you are asked to see him.

How might you proceed regarding this problem?

In the absence of circumstances suggesting other conditions, he probably has an effusion.
Your first task will be to try to determine

- Its cause
- Its effects

How might you try to establish the cause?

Initially, by developing a reasonable differential diagnosis.

How might you do this?

- The insidious development of a large pleural effusion in a previously healthy man is in itself very suggestive of a *malignant process.*
- A careful history relevant to the probable causes of a pleural effusion in such a patient might yield additional information that would influence the differential diagnosis—as shown in Table 15-1.

TABLE 15-1. SCREENING HISTORY IN A PATIENT WITH AN INSIDIOUS ONSET OF A PLEURAL EFFUSION

Source	Finding	Potential significance
Review of systems		
GENERAL HEALTH	Fever	Infection—pneumonia
		Tuberculosis
		Malignant disease
		Pulmonary embolism
		Systemic lupus erythematosus
		(Subphrenic abscess)
		(Amebic hepatitis)
	Sweating	Pulmonary embolism
	Drenching night sweats	Malignant lymphoma
		Tuberculosis

(continued)

Source	Finding	Potential significance
	Weight loss and/or easy fatigability	Malignant disease Tuberculosis Heart failure
RESPIRATORY SYSTEM	Disproportionate dyspnea	Pulmonary embolism Associated atelectasis Heart failure Lymphangitic tumor
	Cough and/or wheezing	Pneumonia Malignant disease Heart failure Pulmonary embolism Tuberculosis
	Hemoptysis	Malignant disease Tuberculosis Pulmonary embolism and infarction
	Pleuritic pain	Pneumonia Pulmonary embolism Systemic lupus erythematosus Tuberculosis Malignant disease
CARDIOVASCULAR SYSTEM	Orthopnea Paroxysmal nocturnal dyspnea Ankle swelling	Heart failure
	Central chest pain	Pulmonary embolism
	Palpitations	Ischemic heart disease, and hence either Heart failure, or Myocardial infarction and Dressler's syndrome
	Syncope	Pulmonary embolism Heart disease and heart failure
	Raynaud's phenomenon	Systemic lupus erythematosus
	Swelling and/or pain in a lower limb	Deep vein thrombosis and pulmonary embolism
MUSCULOSKELETAL SYSTEM	Joint pain or swelling	Systemic lupus erythematosus Malignant disease A drug reaction
SKIN	Photosensitivity Rashes Alopecia	Systemic lupus erythematosus
	Skin lesions or rash	Systemic lupus erythematosus Malignant disease A drug reaction
GASTROINTESTINAL SYSTEM	Abdominal pain or discomfort	A subphrenic abscess Amebic hepatitis Pancreatitis Heart failure

(continued)

TABLE 15-1. SCREENING HISTORY IN A PATIENT WITH AN
INSIDIOUS ONSET OF A PLEURAL EFFUSION *(Continued)*

Source	Finding	Potential significance
	Abdominal distention	Ascites due to cirrhosis of the liver, or the nephrotic syndrome
	Diarrhea, especially if there were blood and/or mucus in the stool	Amebic dysentery Malignant disease of the gastro-intestinal tract
The past history and problem list	Recurrent episodes of pleuritic pain	Systemic lupus erythematosus Pulmonary embolism
	Recurrent bouts of pneumonia	Malignant disease Tuberculosis
	Recent surgery, trauma, immobiliza-tion, bed rest Cerebrovascular ac-cident (or pregnancy)	Pulmonary embolism
	Recent abdominal surgery	Subphrenic abscess
	Recent myocardial infarction	Pulmonary embolism Heart failure Dressler's syndrome
	Recent chest trauma	A traumatic effusion
PRIOR DOCU-MENTATION OF, FOR EXAMPLE:	Heart disease	Heart failure Deep vein thrombosis and pulmonary embolism
	Malignant disease	A malignant effusion A transudate consequent on lymph node obstruction tumor, or possibly due to damage to lymphatic drainage by radiation therapy or surgery Deep vein thrombosis and pulmonary embolism Pericardial tamponade Infection distal to an obstructed bronchus The nephrotic syndrome and hypo-proteinemia
Family history	Tuberculosis in other family members	Tuberculosis
Life situation	Immigration from, or recent travel to, endemic areas	Tuberculosis Amebic hepatitis Coccidioidomycosis
	Occupational exposure to tuberculosis	Tuberculosis

(continued)

TABLE 15-1. SCREENING HISTORY IN A PATIENT WITH AN
INSIDIOUS ONSET OF A PLEURAL EFFUSION *(Continued)*

Source	Finding	Potential significance
	Low socioeconomic status	Tuberculosis
	Exposure to asbestos or other dusts	Mesothelioma Carcinoma of the lung
Alcohol, cigarette and drug exposure	Excessive alcohol consumption	Cirrhosis of the liver Alcoholic cardiomyopathy and cardiac failure Thiamine deficiency and cardiac failure Perhaps an increased propensity to tuberculosis and bronchogenic carcinoma
	Cigarette smoking	Bronchogenic carcinoma
Medications	Use of drugs	Possible "allergic" pleural effusion

*From this initial history you learn that the patient has felt
feverish on several occasions in the past month, that he has had
drenching night sweats on three occasions, and that he has lost
about 10 lbs in weight during this time.*

*He has just returned from a year at Lahore University in India.
As a student he had spent two summers working as a stationary
engineer in a heating plant.*

He smokes 20 cigarettes a day, and has done so for 20 years.

**What constitutes a reasonable differential diagnosis in this man—and
why?**

1. Bronchogenic Carcinoma

It is a common condition, and is rendered even more likely in
this patient by his smoking history, his probable occupational
exposure to asbestos, and the 10-lb weight loss.

2. Tuberculosis

He has just returned from an endemic area, and the associated
symptoms of fever, night sweats, and weight loss are very
suggestive.

3. A Lymphoma

These symptoms of fever, night sweats, and weight loss are also
very suggestive of a lymphoma.

4. Pleural Mesothelioma

His probable exposure to asbestos renders this a very real consideration.

5. Amebic Hepatitis

This might need consideration because of the stay in India, and the fever.

6. Pulmonary Embolism

Because of a long flight, the fever, and its sinister implications if not diagnosed and treated, this possibility must be remembered.

What further points in the history might be of specific diagnostic value?

The **REVIEW OF SYSTEMS** might reveal, with regard to

- Skin
  - A history of pruritus, which would suggest a lymphoma
- Alcohol consumption
  - An area of localized pain precipitated by even a single drink, or by smoking marijuana, which would also suggest a lymphoma.

What findings in the physical examination would be of specific diagnostic value, and what additional features should you be alert to because of their differential diagnostic significance?

With regard to

1. The General Appearance of the Patient

An appearance of "chronic ill-health" would be in keeping with all of the disorders being considered above.

2. Vital Signs

- Fever would similarly be in keeping with all of these conditions.
- A swinging temperature might indicate a subphrenic abscess.
- Hypotension would favor pulmonary embolism, and, as a very "long shot", tuberculosis with hypoadrenalism.

- Hypertension would suggest possible hypertensive heart disease complicated by heart failure; or possibly systemic lupus erythematosus with renal involvement.

3. **The Hand**

- Clubbing of the fingers would strongly favor a bronchogenic malignancy, or possibly a lymphoma.
- Palmar erythema, Dupuytren's contractures, and asterixis would suggest chronic liver disease.

4. **The Head**

- Jaundice would favor involvement of the liver or biliary tree by malignant disease. Amebic hepatitis would be possible, and jaundice would also be consistent with pulmonary embolism. A subphrenic abscess, and chronic liver disease would need to be considered.
- Phlyctenular conjunctivitis would be a rare but highly significant feature of tuberculosis.
- Horner's syndrome would strongly favor bronchogenic carcinoma, or a lymphoma.

5. **The Neck**

- Enlargement of the supraclavicular lymph nodes would strongly favor a bronchogenic carcinoma, and would also support a diagnosis of a lymphoma.
- More extensive cervical adenopathy would favor a lymphoma. Systemic lupus erythematosus and a drug reaction would need consideration.
- Hoarseness would favor malignant disease, with involvement of the recurrent laryngeal nerve. Tuberculous involvement of the vocal cords would need consideration.
- Elevation of the jugular venous pressure might be indicative, in *this* patient, of superior vena caval obstruction or of cardiac tamponade, and hence highly suggestive of malignant disease, and possibly of tuberculous pericarditis. Heart failure would obviously need consideration.
- A giant "a" wave would suggest pulmonary hypertension, and hence pulmonary embolism.

6. **The Thorax**

- There will be the signs of a large effusion.
- If the mediastinum were paradoxically shifted *toward* the

effusion, this might suggest associated atelectases, perhaps resulting from bronchogenic carcinoma.

- Bilateral basal crackles would suggest heart failure
- A pleural friction rub would be consistent with pulmonary embolism, a malignant process, and systemic lupus erythematosus.

7. The Breasts, Axillae, and Chest Wall

- Gynecomastia, spider angiomata, and loss of axillary hair would suggest chronic liver disease.
- Axillary lymphadenopathy would strongly favor a lymphoma. In a female, a mastectomy scar, a breast lump, nipple retraction, or nipple disease would strongly suggest metastatic spread from a breast cancer.

8. The Precordium

- The apex beat might be very prominent—suggestive of heart disease, and hence of heart failure; or difficult to palpate, suggestive of cardiac tamponade, and hence of malignant disease, or possibly of constrictive pericarditis due to tuberculosis.
- A right ventricular lift would favor pulmonary hypertension due to pulmonary embolism, as would a loud pulmonary component of the second heart sound (P2).
- An S3 gallop rhythm would favor heart failure, and might suggest pulmonary embolism.
- The presence of murmurs would suggest underlying heart disease, and hence heart failure.

9. The Abdomen, Scrotum, and Rectum

- Abdominal distention,with evidence of ascites,would favor a diagnosis of malignant disease, but would also raise the possibilities of chronic liver disease, the nephrotic syndrome, constrictive pericarditis, and cardiac failure.
- Subcostal tenderness would suggest a subphrenic abscess.
- Hepatomegaly would further support a diagnosis of malignant disease, both bronchogenic carcinoma *and* lymphoma, but would also be in keeping with amebic hepatitis and constrictive pericarditis. Heart failure and chronic liver disease would again need consideration.
- Splenomegaly would favor a lymphoma, chronic liver disease, and systemic lupus erythematosus.

- Testicular atrophy would suggest chronic liver disease.
- Thickening and irregularity of the epididymis would favor tuberculosis.
- Prostatic hypertrophy and/or nodularity would suggest a primary prostatic malignancy with pleuropulmonary metastases.

10. The Pelvic Organs (in a Woman)

A mass, on vaginal examination, would be very suggestive of malignant disease—especially of an ovary—with pleuropulmonary spread. A Meig's syndrome would also be possible.

11. The Extremities

- Edema of a single limb, especially if associated with tenderness of the limb, would be very much in favor of deep vein thrombosis and pulmonary embolism. Lymphatic obstruction by tumor would also be possible.
- Bilateral leg edema would suggest heart failure, tamponade, constrictive pericarditis, cirrhosis of the liver, and the nephrotic syndrome.
- Erythema nodosum would favor tuberculosis (and would suggest coccidioidomycosis or sarcoidosis).

How should you proceed?

This will depend very much upon the findings actually elicited in the physical examination, and their diagnostic impact.

- If, for example, the patient were noted to have generalized lymphadenopathy and splenomegaly, a lymphoma would be very likely, and the logical step would be to seek confirmation through biopsy of an accessible node.
- Similarly, a single supraclavicular node might reasonably be biopsied, seeking confirmation of a bronchogenic carcinoma, or a lymphoma.
- If the physical examination were noncontributory, further investigations would obviously be indicated, keeping in mind the original differential diagnosis.

Investigations might well include:

- A complete blood count
- Appropriate serum chemistry

- Aspiration of the pleural fluid with analysis as to its
  - Chemistry
  - Cytology
  - Bacteriology, and
  - Hematology
- A pleural biopsy—submitted for histology and culture
- Repeat chest radiograph, after draining the fluid to view the underlying lung
- A tuberculin skin test
- Sputum cytology and appropriate bacteriology
- A lung scan
- A liver scan

It is important to remember that diseases can and do occur in the absence of their usual clinical manifestations. Treatable entities such as pulmonary embolism or tuberculosis, therefore, should not be excluded without very careful consideration, and investigation, if deemed appropriate.

Once the cause for a pleural effusion is established, how should you proceed?

New questions must now be asked, and their nature will depend on the cause for the effusion.

For example: If the effusion were found to be due to malignant disease, it would then be important to decide

- Whether a search for a primary lesion were indicated; and if so, how extensive this search should be.
- Whether there were other evidence of metastatic disease, and how extensively the patient should be investigated in this regard.
- The most appropriate form of management for the malignant process itself.
- Whether the effusion per se requires symptomatic management.

This latter decision would be based to some extent on the answer to the question:

- "What are the effects of the pleural effusion in this man?"

What are the possible effects of a pleural effusion?

- Dyspnea on effort
- Progression to an empyema
- Progression to pleural fibrosis and thickening, with eventual incarceration of the lung and restrictive lung disease—the "trapped lung"

How may the extent of dyspnea on effort be determined?

From a careful history, by determining, as quantitatively as possible, the patient's level of activity. Everyday activities should be assessed to try to discover how much less he is able to do now than in the past.

CHAPTER 16

Jaundice

Jaundice can manifest either as a *symptom*—with the patient noticing, and complaining of, a yellowish discoloration of skin or eyes; or a *sign,* with the physician detecting a characteristic yellow discoloration of a sclerae, skin, or sublingual mucosa. Sometimes it is quite obvious and striking; usually it requires careful and thoughtful observation in a good natural light for its detection.

What "clues" should alert the clinician to look for jaundice?

- Complaints by the patient of
  - A yellowish discoloration of the skin or sclera
  - The passage of dark urine
- The presence of clinical circumstances known to be associated with, or complicated by, the development of jaundice—for example:
  - Alcoholism
  - The administration of certain drugs
  - Recent surgery or blood transfusion
  - Known malignant disease
- Even in the absence of "clues," inspection for jaundice should comprise part of the physical examination.

Does yellowish discoloration of the skin and/or sclera always imply jaundice?

- It usually does, but not *always.* Chloroquine photosensitivity and carotenemia are examples of conditions that may mimic jaundice.

How may jaundice be confirmed?

This requires laboratory testing:

- Urine can be tested for the presence of bilirubin.
- Definite confirmation depends on detecting elevated serum bilirubin levels.

Is an elevated serum bilirubin level always detectable on clinical examination?

No. Clinically detectable jaundice usually demands a serum bilirubin level greater than 2 mg/dl. Where jaundice is suspected, but not detected, laboratory bilirubin assay is indicated.

What is the clinical significance of jaundice and hyperbilirubinemia?

- It may be a clue to underlying significant disease.
- It may reflect the development of complications in the course of a known disease or treatment program.
- In the newborn infant, marked hyperbilirubinemia may produce catastrophic consequences—kernicterus.

Once jaundice is detected and confirmed, how should the clinician proceed?

The clinician should attempt to determine the *cause* of the jaundice in *that particular* patient.

How might you reasonably approach the question of etiology?

You might consider:

- The "associated clinical circumstances" for clues as to likely causes in a particular patient

- The common, and hence likely, causes in the specific population group which the patient represents
- Treatable causes

During your third year rotation in medicine, you are asked to see a 34-year-old woman who has been referred to the Gastroenterology Department because she is jaundiced. Her serum bilirubin level is 5 mg/dl.

How might a review of the PROBLEM LIST influence your thinking about the possible causes for jaundice in this patient?

A previous diagnosis of (for example), *carcinoma of the breast* would suggest that her jaundice might be due to

- Parenchymal liver disease; for example,
  - ○ Metastatic involvement of the liver
  - ○ The hepatotoxic effects of chemotherapeutic agents
  - ○ Viral hepatitis resulting from parenteral therapy
  - ○ The hepatotoxic consequences of sepsis
- Extrahepatic biliary obstruction, caused by tumor compressing and invading the common bile duct
- Hemolysis, perhaps due to disseminated intravascular coagulation

If she had recently undergone *surgery*, jaundice might be due to

- Parenchymal liver disease, resulting from
  - ○ Halothane hepatitis
  - ○ Viral or drug-induced hepatitis
  - ○ The combined effects of hypotension, hypoxemia, and sepsis
- Extrahepatic biliary obstruction due to
  - ○ Bile duct injury

If she were *pregnant,* jaundice would be especially likely to be due to

- Parenchymal liver disease, including
  - ○ Viral hepatitis
  - ○ Recurrent intrahepatic cholestatic jaundice of pregnancy
  - ○ Drug-related hepatitis—tetracycline is especially important in this regard.

If the review of the problem list were not helpful in this patient, it would then be appropriate to consider those conditions most likely to cause jaundice in a young woman.

What are the common, and hence likely, causes for her jaundice?

1. **Parenchymal Liver Disease**
   - Acute hepatitis
     - Viral
     - Alcohol
     - Drug, or
     - Toxin-induced
   - Chronic liver disease
     - Alcohol-related

2. **Obstructive Jaundice**
   - Common bile duct stones

How might you determine which of these causes is indeed responsible?

- By taking a **HISTORY** aimed at detecting the known symptoms of these various disorders, or the features that would indicate one of them.
- By looking very carefully for their characteristic **PHYSICAL SIGNS.**

You should be alert to clues in the history and physical examination to other, and perhaps rarer, causes of jaundice. Those causes of jaundice that might require specific therapy always should receive careful consideration.

What are the "treatable" causes of jaundice?

- Extrahepatic cholestasis (especially if due to common bile duct stones) can almost always be corrected surgically.
- Drug-related hepatitis can usually be cured by discontinuing the responsible drug.
- Alcoholic liver disease: abstinence is usually beneficial, if it can be achieved.

- Hepatotoxins: cure may be possible, if exposure can be avoided.
- Chronic active hepatitis: corticosteroids and immunosuppressive drugs may be of value.
- Weil's disease: antibiotics are indicated.

What might be learned from a STRUCTURED INTERVIEW in this patient?

The **REVIEW OF SYSTEMS** might reveal with regard to

1. Her General Health

- Fever
- Fatigue
- Malaise, lassitude, and weakness

These symptoms would be most characteristic of acute hepatitis. They may occur in the patient with chronic alcoholic liver disease.

- Rigors—most suggestive of biliary obstruction and cholangitis, but possible at the onset of acute hepatitis
- Weight loss—suggestive of chronic alcoholic liver disease, or possibly carcinoma of the pancreas

2. Her Gastrointestinal System

- The characteristic prodromal symptoms of hepatitis:
  - Profound anorexia
  - Distaste for cigarettes
  - Nausea and vomiting
- Features possibly indicative of chronic alcoholism, and hence suggestive of either acute alcoholic hepatitis or chronic liver disease. These include:
  - Morning nausea and anorexia
  - Hematemesis (from a variety of mechanisms, including gastritis, varices, a bleeding diathesis, or Mallory-Weiss syndrome)
- A history of abdominal pain:
  - The patient with gallstones might have had significant attacks of abdominal colic, while the patient with hepatitis might complain of an ache in the right upper quadrant.

○ Epigastric or back pain might suggest a pancreatic carcinoma, as might the absence of pain.

● Abnormalities of bowel habit:

○ Diarrhea is uncommon in these disorders, but would be compatible with both acute hepatitis and chronic alcoholism.

○ Pale stools are common and reflect impaired bile secretion, but have little differential diagnostic significance.

3. **Her Skin**

● A history of pruritus—a symptom indicative of obstruction of bile flow, and hence suggestive of

○ Common bile duct stones

○ Pancreatic carcinoma

○ Primary biliary cirrhosis

○ Other causes for intrahepatic cholestasis

Pruritus is not usually prominent in the patient with acute hepatitis.

Consideration of the **PAST HISTORY** might reveal:

● The possibility of exposure, within the preceding 6 months, to hepatitis virus, via (for example):

○ Blood transfusion

○ Parenteral therapy

○ Tattooing

● Previous gallbladder surgery—which would suggest a common bile duct stone

● Preceding attacks of

○ Abdominal pain

○ Nausea and vomiting

—suggestive of biliary obstruction by stone.

Review of the **LIFE SITUATION** might reveal clues related to

1. **Occupational Hazards**

● Occupational exposure to blood, or blood products, as in a

○ Nurse,

○ Physician

○ Laboratory worker, etc.

would increase the likelihood of viral hepatitis.

- An occupation with exposure to potential hepatotoxins would raise the possibility of acute toxic hepatitis.
- An occupation that is perhaps more likely to be associated with alcoholic excesses (*e.g.,* bartender) or a poor employment record might suggest alcohol-related liver disease.
- An occupation involving employment as
  - A sewage worker or
  - A veterinarian

might suggest Weil's disease.

2. Hobbies, or Other Sources of Exposure to Hepatotoxins

3. Personal Problems

For example,

- Marital problems
- Conflict with the law
- Social maladjustments

would suggest

- Alcohol-related liver disease, or
- Viral hepatitis in a drug addict

as the basis for this patient's jaundice.

With regard to the **MEDICATION HISTORY:** a knowledge of the patient's drug therapy might suggest a drug-related cause for her jaundice.

- Chlorpromazine
- Methyltestosterone
- Phenytoin
- Contraceptive drugs

are among many drugs that are significant in this regard.

With regard to the **HISTORY CONCERNING ALCOHOL, SMOKING, AND DRUG HABITS:**

- A description of the patient's past and present alcohol intake might very usefully point to either acute alcoholic hepatitis or chronic alcoholic liver disease as a cause for her jaundice.
- Drug addiction, particularly "mainlining," is a common antecedent of acute viral hepatitis.

What signs would you specifically look for in the routine PHYSICAL EXAMINATION in trying to differentiate among these common causes for jaundice?

With regard to

1. The General Appearance of the Patient

- A young adult probably has acute hepatitis.
- The characteristic facies and appearance of the alcoholic would be significant.

2. Vital Signs

- *Fever* can occur in any of these conditions, but if high and labile, would favor gallstones with cholangitis, or perhaps an intra-abdominal abscess (which sometimes produces cholestatic jaundice).

3. Mental Status

- Features of hepatic encephalopathy would suggest either severe acute hepatitis or chronic liver disease.
- Dementia, Korsakoff's psychosis, delirium tremens, etc., would suggest chronic alcoholic liver disease.

4. The Hand

- Palmar erythema
- Dupuytren's contractures
- Whiteness of the nails

—would be evidence of chronic liver disease.

- Asterixis would suggest either chronic liver disease or severe acute hepatitis.
- Clubbing of the fingers might suggest primary biliary cirrhosis.

5. The Head and Neck

- Fetor hepaticus would suggest either chronic liver disease or fulminating acute hepatitis.
- Parotid enlargement would suggest chronic alcoholic liver disease.

6. Skin Changes

- Bruising is frequent in the jaundiced subject, but has little differential diagnostic value.

- Spider angiomata would point to chronic liver disease—especially alcoholic liver disease.
- Scratch marks would suggest cholestasis.
- A petechial rash might suggest Weil's disease.
- Xanthomas and xanthelasmata would suggest primary biliary cirrhosis, or other long-standing cholestatic processes.

7. The Thorax

- Gynecomastia, and
- Loss of axillary hair

might suggest chronic liver disease, especially alcoholic liver disease.

8. Abdomen and Scrotum

Findings in the abdomen might suggest acute hepatitis, chronic liver disease, or gallstones:

- Acute hepatitis would be suggested by
  - Tenderness to palpation or percussion over the liver
  - Slight or moderate hepatomegaly
  - Slight splenomegaly
- Chronic liver disease would be suggested by
  - A female escutcheon (in a male)
  - Abdominal distention due to ascites
  - Firm hepatomegaly, or a marked reduction in liver size
  - Significant and firm splenomegaly
  - Testicular atrophy (in a male)
- Choledocholithiasis would be suggested by
  - Tender hepatomegaly—if ascending cholangitis has developed

In addition:

- A palpable gallbladder would suggest a pancreatic carcinoma (Courvoisier's law).
- An abdominal mass or tenderness, perinephric tenderness, or a rectal mass and tenderness would all suggest an intra-abdominal abscess as a possible cause for cholestatic jaundice.

9. The Extremities

- Evidence of a peripheral neuropathy would suggest chronic alcoholic liver disease.

Are there other causes for jaundice that should be considered?

A hemolytic process, and Gilbert's disease, are sufficiently common to warrant consideration, in most patients whose jaundice is only minimal.

What features would suggest hemolysis?

With regard to

1. The History

- Symptoms often date back many years, even to childhood. The patient may admit to the passage of dark urine, and to easy fatigability.
- There might be prior documentation of a hemolytic process or of diseases known to be complicated by the development of hemolysis.
- There might be a family history of hemolytic anemia, splenectomy, or cholecystectomy.

2. The Physical Examination

- Pallor and/or
- Splenomegaly

would be very suggestive of hemolysis.

3. Routine Hematologic Studies

- Reticulocytosis is especially significant.
- It is important to remember that hemoglobin concentration is variable and may be normal in hemolysis.
- Conversely, anemia could complicate many of the diseases manifesting jaundice, where hemolysis is not a factor.

What features suggest Gilbert's disease?

This disorder comprises a diagnosis of exclusion in those patients with mild unconjugated hyperbilirubinemia in whom occult or compensated hemolysis has been carefully excluded.

Upon further evaluation of your patient, you learn that she is a prisoner at a local penitentiary.
She was well until 1 week ago, when she developed anorexia and

some right upper quadrant discomfort. She was nauseated and had vomited several times, but is now beginning to feel better.
A fellow prisoner noticed 2 days ago that she was "yellow."
Physical examination reveals moderate, slightly tender hepatomegaly, but she is otherwise normal.

What is the most likely diagnosis?

- Viral hepatitis

What investigations are indicated?

- Determination of the serum bilirubin and SGOT concentrations
- Follow-up in 1 week

CHAPTER 17

Splenomegaly

A palpable mass in the left upper quadrant is a common physical finding. Before automatically assuming that it represents splenomegaly, and therefore launching a campaign to determine the cause and effects of the splenomegaly, it is always worth reflecting, if only for moment, that such a mass might have a different basis.

What are the conditions that might readily mimic the physical signs of splenomegaly?

- A renal mass
- A pancreatic pseudocyst
- A mass in or around the splenic flexure of the colon
- An enlarged left lobe of the liver
- An adrenal mass
- A retroperitoneal mass
- An omental mass

What findings on physical examination are pathognomonic of splenomegaly?

There are no findings pathognomonic of splenomegaly!

What are the signs that on further examination of the mass render splenomegaly more probable?

- An enlarged spleen is often fairly "superficial," and best felt with light and gentle palpation. A renal mass tends to be more posterior and deeper, and requires firmer, or bimanual, palpation to feel. A liver mass also is better felt on firmer palpation.

- An enlarged spleen passes upward beneath the rib margin, and its upper edge cannot be palpated. A colonic mass can sometimes be palpated in its entirety.
- The spleen usually enlarges in a downward and *medial* direction, while a renal mass is usually more lateral.
- An enlarged spleen moves well with respiration—downward and medially. A renal mass moves in a more vertical manner.
- With splenic enlargement, dullness to percussion over the left lower chest *persists* with deep inspiration, while the sound often becomes resonant with a renal mass.

Does palpating a "splenic notch" have relevance?

No. The notch is not always palpable in an enlarged spleen. Conversely, a notch may be mimicked in many of the masses listed above.

How might the remainder of the physical examination contribute to the diagnosis?

If other features present indicate disease states in which splenomegaly might be *anticipated,* this would certainly increase the probability that a left upper quadrant mass is the result of an enlarged spleen—as, for example, in the patient with

- Generalized lymphadenopathy
- Features of chronic liver disease
- Evidence of a blood dyscrasia

Conversely, gastrointestinal symptoms or known gastrointestinal disease would increase the likelihood of a gastric, pancreatic, or colonic mass; genitourinary symptoms, or known renal disease, or a family history of polycystic kidneys, would increase the probability of a renal mass; evidence of Cushing's syndrome might suggest an adrenal mass, etc.

Are further confirmatory investigations indicated?

- An abdominal radiograph is useful for estimating spleen size.

- A liver and spleen scan may be very valuable in estimating size.

Either or both of these studies should be readily employed where doubt exists as to the nature of the left upper quadrant mass. Once the presence of splenomegaly is confirmed as definitively as is reasonable or appropriate, the usual two questions should be posed:

- Why does this patient have splenomegaly?
- What are its possible consequences, and are they evident?

The approach to the etiology of splenomegaly will vary considerably according to whether this finding is encountered in

- An otherwise entirely healthy patient
- A chronically ill patient
- An acutely ill patient

SPLENOMEGALY IN A "WELL" PATIENT

In the course of learning how to examine the abdomen, you are asked to palpate the abdomen of one of your 23-year-old colleagues. To your absolute amazement, you detect a mass in his left upper quadrant that has all the characteristics of an enlarged spleen.

How should you proceed?

The most likely explanation for an asymptomatic left upper quadrant mass in a healthy medical student is indeed splenomegaly.

Many of the disorders causing asymptomatic splenomegaly are capable of detection without invasive, or even radiologic, investigation.

It is thus quite reasonable to interview and examine him, and to do preliminary blood studies on the assumption that he does indeed have splenomegaly.

Should an explanation for splenomegaly not be rapidly forthcoming, then investigations should be undertaken to confirm the splenic nature of the mass before proceeding further.

What causes for splenomegaly might reasonably be considered in this student?

- A variety of hematologic disorders:

○ Hemolytic anemias
○ Chronic myeloid leukemia
○ Essential thrombocythemia
○ Acute leukemia
○ A lymphoma
• Congestive splenomegaly, due to
○ Portal or splenic vein thrombosis
• Splenic infiltrates
○ Splenic cyst
○ Gaucher's disease
○ Sarcoidosis
• Chronic infections
○ Malaria
• Idiopathic splenomegaly

How might the HISTORY help to establish the cause of your colleague's splenomegaly?

The **PAST HISTORY** might reveal

• Previous documentation of one of the above disorders
• Periumbilical sepsis, or umbilical vein catheterization in the neonatal period—suggestive of portal vein thrombosis
• Episodes of jaundice, or biliary colic, suggestive of a hemolytic process
• Episodes of bone pain—suggestive of Gaucher's disease

The **FAMILY HISTORY** might reveal

• Ethnic origin in Southeast Asia, rendering alpha thalassemia more likely; in the Mediterranean countries, with beta thalassemia a consequent possibility; or in Africa, which is perhaps suggestive of other hemoglobinopathies
• Documentation of hereditary spherocytosis, or a hemoglobinopathy in other family members; or of Gaucher's disease in siblings—with obvious diagnostic implications
• Documentation of jaundice or biliary tract disease; or the need for splenectomy in other family members—factors that would suggest an inherited hemolytic process

The **LIFE SITUATION** might reveal

• Origin in, or travel to, Africa, South America, or Southeast

Asia, which would increase the probability of malaria, schistosomiasis (or even kala-azar!)

- Exposure to unpasteurized milk, suggesting brucellosis

What might be learned from the PHYSICAL EXAMINATION?

This might reveal, with regard to

1. The Head and Neck

- Pallor—suggestive of anemia and a hematologic disease
- Jaundice—suggestive of a hemolytic process
- Brown pingueculae in the sclera—suggestive of Gaucher's disease
- Lymphadenopathy—suggestive of a leukemic or lymphomatous process; or sarcoidosis

2. The Thorax and Axillae

- Lymphadenopathy—with implications as above
- Sternal tenderness—suggestive of acute leukemia

3. The Abdomen

- Hepatomegaly and/or inguinal lymphadenopathy, again suggestive of leukemia, lymphoma, or sarcoidosis

4. The Skin

- Skin lesions suggestive of sarcoidosis—papules, nodules, or plaques in the skin of the face, particularly
- Skin pigmentation suggestive of Gaucher's disease—brownish yellow pigmentation of the head, neck, hands, and lower legs

What investigations are indicated?

- A complete blood count, including very careful inspection of the blood film
- Possibly hemoglobin electrophoresis and an osmotic fragility test
- A chest radiograph
- A marrow aspirate, if leukemia or Gaucher's disease were serious considerations
- Lymph node biopsy, if significant adenopathy were evident

If a diagnosis were not established, how would you proceed?

- To a flat radiograph of the abdomen and a liver and spleen scan, to confirm the nature of the mass.
- If splenomegaly were indeed confirmed, observation every 6 months for a while might be indicated in this asymptomatic subject.
- If splenomegaly were *not* confirmed, investigation as to the nature of the mass would be strongly indicated.

SPLENOMEGALY IN A CHRONICALLY ILL SUBJECT

During a "clinical diagnosis" session, you see a 65-year-old man who has felt generally unwell for the past 6 months. During this time he has been feverish, on occasion. He has been tired and lacking in energy, and has lost about 10 lbs in weight. He looks "chronically ill."

The patient had been seen in the outpatient clinic, where moderate splenomegaly was noted. This was confirmed by both abdominal radiograph and liver and spleen scan.

He has been admitted to the hospital "for investigation."

How might you approach this problem?

The splenomegaly and the systemic symptoms may quite clearly be unrelated. It is possible that a patient with hereditary spherocytosis and splenomegaly may develop a carcinoma of the lung, with systemic symptoms of that disorder. Nevertheless, simple logic dictates as a first step, that these manifestations be grouped, and that you then develop a differential diagnosis with respect to those disorders likely to manifest both splenomegaly and general ill health.

What are the disorders that might manifest both splenomegaly and general ill health?

1. Congestive Splenomegaly

Possible causes are

- Cirrhosis of the liver
- Portal or splenic vein occlusion
- Hepatic vein occlusion

2. Hematologic Diseases

- The chronic myeloproliferative diseases
  - Polycythemia vera
  - Essential thrombocythemia
  - Myelofibrosis
  - Chronic myeloid leukemia
- Chronic lymphocytic leukemia
- The lymphomas and their variants
- Autoimmune hemolytic anemia
- Acute leukemia

3. Subacute and Chronic Infections

- Histoplasmosis
- Brucellosis
- Tuberculosis
- Bacterial endocarditis
- Malaria
- Schistosomiasis
- Leishmaniasis (kala-azar)

4. Collagen-vascular Diseases

- Felty's syndrome
- Systemic lupus erythematosus (SLE)

5. Miscellaneous

- Sarcoidosis
- Idiopathic splenomegaly

How might the HISTORY help in differentiating among these various disorders?

The **REVIEW OF SYSTEMS** might reveal the following symptoms, with regard to

1. His General Health

- Drenching night sweats—perhaps suggestive of lymphoma, tuberculosis, or histoplasmosis

2. His Skin

- Pruritus—suggestive of polycythemia vera or lymphoma

- A rash—suggestive of acute leukemia, a lymphoma, endocarditis, sarcoidosis, or SLE
- Photosensitivity—suggestive of SLE
- Bruising—suggestive of liver disease, or leukemia

3. **The Musculoskeletal System**

- Polyarthralgia—suggestive of rheumatoid arthritis and Felty's syndrome, SLE, a lymphoma, sarcoidosis, or endocarditis

4. **The Respiratory System**

- Pleuritic chest pain—suggestive of SLE
- Cough—suggestive of tuberculosis
- Dyspnea—suggestive of lymphoma, sarcoidosis, or SLE

5. **The Cardiovascular System**

- Raynaud's phenomenon—suggestive of SLE
- Intermittent claudication, coldness, and numbness of the feet—suggestive of peripheral vascular disease, and hence polycythemia vera, or essential thrombocythemia
- Painful fingers or toes, or erythromelalgia—also suggestive of these disorders
- A painful, swollen leg—suggestive of deep vein thrombosis and, again, the chronic myeloproliferative disorders

6. **The Central Nervous System**

- Transient ischemic attacks—possibly indicative of a myeloproliferative disorder

7. **The Gastrointestinal System**

- Hematemesis and/or melena—suggestive of esophageal varices and chronic liver disease

A review of the **PROBLEM LIST** or **PAST HISTORY** might reveal (for example):

- Prior documentation of one of these disorders. Tuberculosis might have been diagnosed many years previously.
- Previous documentation of rheumatic fever—which might now be complicated by endocarditis
- Recent dental work or urethral instrumentation—with the potential for the subsequent development of endocarditis
- Known alcoholism—suggestive now of cirrhosis of the liver

- Rheumatoid arthritis, now possibly complicated by progression to Felty's syndrome

A review of the **LIFE SITUATION** might well prove especially valuable in providing a diagnostic lead:

- Occupational history:
  - Work in the health or allied professions might be associated with exposure to tuberculosis or brucellosis
  - Dairy farmers, goatherds, meat packers, abattoir workers, and veterinarians might be especially susceptible to brucellosis.
- Travel out of the country might predispose to the tropical diseases.

How might the PHYSICAL EXAMINATION contribute to the differential diagnosis?

Within the context of the routine physical examination, it would be important to look for several specific findings, and to be aware of their diagnostic implications. These are listed in Table 17-1.

TABLE 17-1. PHYSICAL FINDINGS OF POTENTIAL DIAGNOSTIC VALUE IN THE PATIENT WITH "CHRONIC ILL HEALTH" AND SPLENOMEGALY

Source	Sign	Potential significance
Pulse	Abnormal character	Possible valvular heart disease—and hence superimposed endocarditis
Hand	Clubbing	
	Osler's nodes	Endocarditis
	Janeway spots	
	Splinter hemorrhages	Endocarditis
		Acute leukemia
		Polycythemia vera
		Essential thrombocythemia
	Palmar erythema	Chronic liver disease
		Polycythemia vera
		Chronic lymphocytic leukemia
		Other lymphomas
	Dupuytren's contractures	Chronic liver disease
	Periungual erythema and telangiectases	SLE
	Digital ulceration	SLE
		Myeloproliferative disease
	Rheumatoid changes	Felty's syndrome

(continued)

TABLE 17-1. PHYSICAL FINDINGS OF POTENTIAL DIAGNOSTIC VALUE IN THE PATIENT WITH "CHRONIC ILL HEALTH" AND SPLENOMEGALY *(Continued)*

Source	Sign	Potential significance
Skin	Petechiae	Acute leukemia
	Bruising	Endocarditis
		SLE
		Polycythemia vera
		Chronic liver disease
	Cutaneous plaques or nodules	Sarcoidosis
	Telangiectases	Chronic liver disease
Head and neck	Jaundice	Chronic liver disease
		A hemolytic anemia
	Pallor	Acute leukemia
		Hemolytic anemia
		Endocarditis
		SLE
	Plethora	Polycythemia vera
Fundus	Venous distention	Polycythemia vera
	Cytoid bodies	SLE
	Roth spots	Endocarditis
	Hemorrhages	Leukemia
Neck	Parotid enlargement	Chronic liver disease
		A lymphoma
	Adenopathy	A lymphoma
		Chronic lymphocytic leukemia
		Acute leukemia
		Sarcoidosis
		SLE
		Brucellosis
		Histoplasmosis
	Abnormalities of the jugular venous pulse	Valvular heart disease, and hence endocarditis
Thorax and axillae	Gynecomastia	Chronic liver disease
	Loss of axillary hair	
	A pleural friction rub	SLE
	Adenopathy	As above
Precordium	Displacement of the apex beat	
	Abnormal pulsations, thrills	
	Abnormalities of the heart sounds	
	Murmurs	Endocarditis
	A pericardial friction rub	Endocarditis
		SLE
Abdomen	Distention—due to ascites	Chronic liver disease
	Hepatomegaly	Chronic liver disease

(continued)

TABLE 17-1. PHYSICAL FINDINGS OF POTENTIAL DIAGNOSTIC
VALUE IN THE PATIENT WITH "CHRONIC ILL HEALTH" AND
SPLENOMEGALY *(Continued)*

Source	Sign	Potential significance
		Lymphoma
		Chronic leukemia
		Myelofibrosis
		Sarcoidosis
		Histoplasmosis
Scrotum	Thickening of deferens	Tuberculosis
	Testicular atrophy	Chronic liver disease
Extremities	Signs of an upper motor neuron lesion	Embolic effects of endocarditis
	A peripheral neuropathy	SLE
		Chronic alcoholic liver disease
	Polyarthritis	Felty's syndrome
		SLE
		Sarcoidosis
	Erythema nodosum	Histoplasmosis

*Upon further evaluation of your patient you learn that he had
prostatic surgery 6 months previously.*

*Physical examination confirms the fever and reveals slight
clubbing of the fingers, but is otherwise unremarkable.*

What is the probable diagnosis?

- Bacterial endocarditis

How should you proceed?

- To a very careful re-evaluation of the physical findings,
  looking for additional supportive evidence of bacterial endocarditis
- To repeated blood cultures and other laboratory investigations in an attempt to confirm this diagnosis

SPLENOMEGALY IN AN ACUTELY ILL PATIENT

*A 24-year-old female patient comes to the Emergency Room
with complaints that she has been "off color" for the past 1-2*

weeks, and that she has been feverish with profound malaise and lassitude over the past 2 days.
   The chief resident sees her briefly, and mentions to you that her spleen is enlarged.
   He asks you to evaluate her in more detail.

How should you proceed?

Again, as in the previous patient, the acute illness and the splenomegaly may be coincidental, but wisdom would again dictate that these features be grouped.

What disorders might then reasonably be considered to account for her illness?

1. Infections

- Infectious mononucleosis (IM) and viral hepatitis (VH) are common and probable.
- Endocarditis is a critical possibility.
- Other infections are possible, and their likelihood will increase in certain circumstances. These disorders include:
  - Brucellosis
  - Cytomegalovirus infection (CMV)
  - Typhoid and paratyphoid infections
  - Rickettsial infections
  - Toxoplasmosis
  - Malaria
  - Secondary syphilis

2. Acute Leukemia

3. Systemic Lupus Erythematosus

These illnesses tend to have many features in common: fever, chills, malaise, lassitude, fatigue, myalgia, anorexia, nausea, headache, cough, and a skin rash.

How might the HISTORY help in their differentiation?

The **REVIEW OF SYSTEMS** might reveal the following symptoms, with regard to

1. **The Gastrointestinal Tract**

   - Profound anorexia and (in a smoker) distaste for cigarettes —suggestive of hepatitis
   - Diarrhea (or constipation)—suggestive of typhoid or para-typhoid fever, especially if blood were present in the stool
   - Jaundice, suggestive of VH or IM

2. **The Eyes, Ears, Nose, and Throat**

   - A severe sore throat—suggestive of IM and also of acute leukemia

3. **The Respiratory System**

   - Pleuritic pain—suggestive of SLE

4. **The Cardiovascular System**

   - Raynaud's phenomenon—suggestive of SLE

5. **The Musculoskeletal System**

   - Joint pains—suggestive of SLE, acute leukemia, VH, or endocarditis

6. **The Central Nervous System**

   - Very severe headache—suggestive of a rickettsial infection
   - Focal neurologic symptoms—suggestive of endocarditis or SLE

7. **The Skin and Hair**

   - Photosensitivity—suggestive of SLE
   - Alopecia—suggestive of SLE and secondary syphilis

A review of the **PAST HISTORY** or **PROBLEM LIST** might reveal

- Possible exposure to blood or blood products in the previous 6 months—which would very much suggest VH
- Recent blood transfusion—suggesting, in addition, CMV (or even possibly malaria)
- Evidence of an immunosuppressed state—rendering CMV or toxoplasmosis more possible
- Previous rheumatic fever—thus increasing the possibility of endocarditis

A **REVIEW OF THE LIFE SITUATION** might reveal

- Specific Occupational Hazards
  - A meat packer would be at risk for brucellosis; and contact with livestock would also suggest Q fever.
  - Veterinarians and laboratory workers are more exposed to the more exotic infections.
  - Medical personnel are especially likely to contract VH.
- A recent camping trip or travel to an endemic area (Southeastern states)—suggestive of a rickettsial infection
- Travel to Asia, Africa, or Latin America—suggestive of malaria
- Exposure to the drug subculture—suggestive of VH or endocarditis
- Ingestion of unpasteurized milk—suggestive of brucellosis
- Potential venereal exposure—suggestive of secondary syphilis
- Known local epidemics—with obvious diagnostic implications

How might the PHYSICAL EXAMINATION help?

With regard to

1. **Vital Signs**
   - A "slow" pulse—slower than might have been anticipated from the temperature, would be suggestive of typhoid fever or a rickettsial illness.
   - Hypotension would suggest a septicemic illness.

2. **Mental Status**
   - Altered consciousness—drowsiness or delirium—would be most suggestive of endocarditis, SLE, or typhoid.

3. **The Skin.** Most of these illnesses can manifest a rash of one form or another:
   - A petechial rash would be most suggestive of leukemia, endocarditis, or SLE, but could also occur in IM, the rickettsial infections, or VH.
   - A maculopapular rash would suggest
     - Typhoid fever, if the rash were especially evident over the upper abdomen
     - A rickettsial infection, especially if there were involve-

ment of the palms and soles—features which would also very strongly suggest syphilis, or toxoplasmosis

- A pustular rash should make one very suspicious of septicemia and endocarditis.
- Urticaria might favor SLE or hepatitis.

4. **The Hand**

- Clubbing, if present, would suggest endocarditis, as would Osler's nodes and Janeway spots.
- Splinter hemorrhages in the fingernails would suggest endocarditis or leukemia.
- Ulceration of the fingertips, and periungual erythema or telangectasia, would favor SLE.
- A rash on the palms would suggest syphilis or a rickettsial infection.

5. **The Head and Neck**

- Jaundice would suggest mononucleosis or hepatitis.
- Puffiness of the eyelids (Hoagland's sign) would suggest IM.
- Pallor would suggest acute leukemia.
- Fundal hemorrhages would suggest acute leukemia or endocarditis, while cytoid bodies would be suggestive of SLE.
- Gum hypertrophy would suggest acute leukemia.
- A faucial membrane would suggest IM or acute leukemia.
- A palatal enanthem would suggest IM.
- Mucous patches would suggest syphilis.
- Cranial nerve palsies might indicate endocarditis, or SLE.
- Cervical adenopathy would suggest IM, acute leukemia, SLE, also brucellosis, toxoplasmosis, CMV, and secondary syphilis.

6. **The Thorax and Axillae**

- A pleural friction rub would suggest SLE.

7. **The Precordium**

- Abnormalities of the heart sounds and the presence or development of murmurs would strongly suggest endocarditis.
- A pericardial friction rub would suggest SLE or endocarditis.

8. The Abdomen

- Hepatomegaly would suggest VH, IM, or leukemia

9. The Rectal Examination

- Condylomata would suggest syphilis.

10. The Extremities

- Peripheral neuropathy would suggest SLE.
- Upper motor neuron pathology would suggest endocarditis.
- Polyarthritis would suggest SLE or endocarditis.

What laboratory studies are indicated?

- A complete blood count
- Urinalysis
- Blood cultures
- A mononucleosis spot test

Other laboratory studies will be dictated by the clinical probabilities and the results of the initial laboratory studies.

In the course of the history and physical examination, you learn that your patient has recently developed Raynaud's phenomenon and that she has had several episodes, lasting 1-2 days, of moderately severe pleuritic pain. Presently she has pain in several of the joints of both hands.

She has generalized lymphadenopathy, and a pericardial friction rub is audible.

What is the most likely diagnosis?

- Systemic lupus erythematosus

How should you proceed?

- To laboratory studies that will confirm this diagnosis
- To a consideration of the possible effects of SLE
- To a decision as to treatment

EFFECTS OF SPLENOMEGALY

What are the potential effects of splenomegaly?

- Local Effects
  - Left upper quadrant discomfort
  - Early satiety
  - Splenic infarction—left upper quadrant pain, possibly referred to the left shoulder, and pleuritic in character
  - Splenic rupture—with massive intraperitoneal bleeding, and shock
- Hematologic effects
  - Anemia
  - Neutropenia, and
  - Thrombocytopenia

By and large these effects are mild, and detectable only on laboratory testing.

The neutropenia may be more profound and may lead to recurrent infections.

CHAPTER 18

Peripheral Edema

Peripheral edema is a common clinical finding, and one that is often the first clue to significant underlying disease.

Once edema has been detected, the initial diagnostic problem is in differentiating between a local cause for the edema and a systemic disease resulting in generalized edema.

How may one decide whether the cause is local or systemic?

This is usually fairly easy, although on occasion it may be difficult. The decision will depend upon

- The distribution of the edema
- Associated clinical features

1. Distribution

- Edema of a single limb usually reflects local pathology.
- Bilateral limb edema is indicative of a systemic disease, but could be due to
  ○ Bilateral varicosities
  ○ Bilateral deep vein pathology
  ○ Bilateral inguinal or pelvic node pathology
  ○ Inferior vena caval obstruction
- A gravitational shift in the distribution of the fluid—involving the ankles and legs, while the patient is ambulatory, and the sacrum when he is confined to bed—would strongly favor a systemic cause.

2. Associated Features

Associated inflammatory features (warmth, tenderness, redness) would suggest local pathology, as would pathology in the region of the draining lymph nodes.

Conversely, accumulation of fluid in potential spaces (ascites, a pleural effusion), or at other sites (eyelids, sacrum) would suggest a systemic process, as would the documentation of disorders known to be associated with generalized edema. The patient with cardiac failure (a systemic disorder) is, however, eminently likely to develop deep vein thrombosis, with unilateral localized edema on this basis.

During your Family Practice internship, while working in a general practitioner's office you see a 27-year-old woman whose presenting complaints are that she has gained about 8 lbs recently and that her feet swell quite markedly toward the end of the day.

There has been no pain, warmth, or discoloration associated with the swelling.

Even a superficial inspection of the patient's feet during the interview shows them to be significantly swollen, and palpation confirms the presence of pitting edema to the level of her knees. You believe that she has generalized edema.

What disease processes should be considered in this patient?

While many exist, it is worthwhile to begin by considering certain common causes of generalized edema. These are:

- Heart failure
- Pericardial tamponade or constrictive pericarditis
- Acute glomerulonephritis
- The nephrotic syndrome
- Chronic liver disease
- Hypoalbuminemia from any cause
- Cyclic edema of females
- Medications

How might a review of the PROBLEM LIST contribute to the differential diagnosis?

Prior documentation of (for example):

1. **Tuberculosis**—would increase the probability of

- Constrictive pericarditis

2. **Malignant disease**—would suggest the possibility of:
- Pericardial tamponade
- Constrictive pericarditis
- Heart failure
- The nephrotic syndrome
- Inferior vena caval obstruction

In the absence of such specific clues, how might you reasonably structure the interview to try to determine which of the more common systemic causes is the cause of this patient's edema?

With regard to the **SYSTEMS REVIEW** relevant to the

1. Cardiovascular System

Complaints of

- Dyspnea on effort
- Orthopnea
- Paroxysmal nocturnal dyspnea

would suggest heart failure as the cause for her edema.

Complaints of

- Palpitations
- Ischemic chest pain (angina pectoris)
- Syncope

would be suggestive of cardiac disease, and hence would also increase the possibility that heart failure is responsible.

2. Genitourinary System

- Altered character of the urine would suggest a diagnosis of
  - Glomerulonephritis

3. Gastrointestinal System

A complaint of

- Jaundice would suggest
  - Liver disease
- Abnormal bowel habits might be indicative of
  - A malabsorption syndrome
  - A protein-losing enteropathy

—disorders that might result in hypoalbuminemia.

4. Medication History

Drugs such as

- Estrogens or prednisone might cause salt and water retention with resultant edema.

With regard to the **PAST HISTORY,** questioning should be directed very specifically to seeking prior documentation of

- Heart disease
- Hypertension

Either of these conditions would suggest

  ○ Heart failure

as the cause for the patient's edema.

- Renal disease, which would suggest
  ○ The nephrotic syndrome
  ○ Heart failure
- Liver disease, or
- Gastrointestinal pathology

which might suggest consequent

  ○ Hypoalbuminemia
- A cyclical pattern

which would favor

  ○ Cyclical edema of females

With regard to the **LIFE SITUATION,** alcohol excesses would suggest

- Chronic liver disease or
- Alcoholic cardiomyopathy

as the basis for this patient's edema.

How might the PHYSICAL EXAMINATION aid in the differential diagnosis?

A routine physical examination seeking the signs listed in Table 18-1 might yield significant diagnostic information.

This examination might also serve to confirm a diagnosis suggested by the history.

TABLE 18-1. PHYSICAL FINDINGS OF POTENTIAL DIAGNOSTIC SIGNIFICANCE IN A PATIENT WITH GENERALIZED EDEMA

Source	Finding	Potential significance
Vital signs		
PULSE	Tachycardia Pulsus alternans	Heart failure
	Pulsus paradoxus	Pericardial disease
BLOOD PRESSURE	Hypertension	Heart failure Glomerulonephritis
Hand	Leukonychia	Hypoalbuminemia
	Palmar erythema	Chronic liver disease
	Dupuytren's contractures	
	Asterixis	
Mental status	Abnormal: Drowsy, confused, disoriented	Chronic liver disease Glomerulonephritis
Head	Fetor hepaticus Jaundice Parotid enlargement	Chronic liver disease
Neck	Elevated jugular venous pressure	Heart failure Pericardial disease Glomerulonephritis
	Kussmaul's sign Rapid Y descent	Pericardial disease
Chest	Spider angiomata Gynecomastia	Chronic liver disease
	Pleural effusion	No differential significance; to be anticipated in a patient with edema
	Ewart's sign (bronchial breathing below the left scapula)	Pericardial tamponade
	Basal crepitations	Heart failure
Precordium	Inability to locate the apex beat	Possible pericardial disease
	Abnormal position or character of the apex beat Murmurs	Heart disease, and hence an in- creased liability to heart failure
	Muffled heart sounds A pericardial friction rub	Pericardial effusion and perhaps tamponade
	A gallop rhythm	Heart failure
Abdomen	Ascites	This is to be anticipated in a patient with generalized edema. If a pre- dominant feature, it would suggest chronic liver disease

What laboratory studies are indicated?

- Urinalysis—seeking evidence of
  - Proteinuria and/or
  - An abnormal sediment
- Serum chemistry
  - Albumin, bilirubin, SGOT, BUN, creatinine, and cholesterol concentrations
- Chest radiograph

Upon further evaluation of your patient, you learn that she has developed increasing dyspnea on effort over the preceding 2 months; and that she has "two-pillow" orthopnea, whereas previously she had used only a single pillow for comfort.

What diagnosis is suggested by the constellation of effort dyspnea, orthopnea, and peripheral edema?

- Congestive heart failure

What physical findings would support this diagnosis—in a patient with leg edema?

With regard to

- The pulse
  - Tachycardia
  - A diminished pulse volume
  - Pulsus alternans
- The neck
  - An elevated jugular venous pressure
- The precordium
  - A gallop rhythm
- The lung fields
  - Bilateral basal crepitations
  - Pleural effusion(s)
- The abdomen
  - Hepatomegaly
  - Ascites

If heart failure is confirmed, how should you proceed?

While you may feel legitimately proud of your progress to this point, the degree of problem resolution is not such that the task has been completed.

The initial question ("Why does this patient have edema?") has received the answer, "Because she is in heart failure." This raises the question, "Why is she in heart failure?" To answer this question demands a knowledge of the causes of heart failure, and an approach that will enable you to differentiate among them— the subject of the next chapter.

CHAPTER 19

Heart Failure

What are the probable causes of heart failure?

These may more easily be considered by conceiving of the heart as a pump, composed of

- The myocardium
- A vascular supply
- A conducting system, and
- Valves

The heart pumps

- Blood

against resistance, in the

- Systemic circulation and the
- Pulmonary circulation

Disease in any part of the system can result in heart failure, as shown in Table 19-1.

TABLE 19-1. ANATOMICAL BASIS OF HEART FAILURE

Site	Disease
Myocardium	Cardiomyopathy
	Myocarditis
	Structural defects
Vascular supply	Ischemic heart disease*
Conducting system	Arrhythmias
Valves	Valvular heart disease
Blood	Too little—anemia
	Too viscous—hyperviscosity
Systemic circulation	Too much resistance—hypertension*
	Too little resistance—high output failure
Pulmonary circulation	Cor pulmonale

*One of the most common causes of heart failure

How might you attempt to differentiate among these disorders?

- By seeking their various characteristic abnormalities in the history, physical examination, and laboratory data
- By seeking or recognizing features which are likely to be associated with one or another of these disorders, and which will therefore increase the likelihood of its presence

DIAGNOSTIC APPROACH TO THE PATIENT IN HEART FAILURE

In addition to trying to determine the basic cause of the congestive failure, it is also important to consider and detect, if possible, the presence of precipitating or aggravating factors that will contribute to heart failure if a predisposing condition already exists.

Table 19-2 lists an orderly approach to evaluating the patient with congestive heart failure, indicating the areas in which information might be sought, and the nature and potential diagnostic significance of the information gathered.

TABLE 19-2. INFORMATION OF POTENTIAL DIAGNOSTIC VALUE IN DETERMINING THE CAUSE OF CONGESTIVE HEART FAILURE

Source	Symptom	Potential Significance
Review of systems Cardiovascular system	Ischemic chest pain: Angina pectoris	Atherosclerotic heart disease
		Valvular heart disease
		Anemia—usually an aggravating rather than a causative, factor
	Myocardial infarction	Precipitation of cardiac failure
	Palpitations	An arrhythmia—rarely a primary factor; usually an aggravating or precipitating factor, and often implying:
		Ischemic heart disease, hypertensive heart disease, valvular heart disease, thyrotoxicosis, or digitalis toxicity as the responsible mechanism for the heart failure
	Pain or swelling of a lower limb	Recurrent emboli—resulting in pulmonary hypertension and cor pulmonale

Source	Symptom	Potential Significance
		Precipitation or aggravation of failure by an embolus
Respiratory system	Chronic or recurrent cough and sputum production; wheezing	Chronic obstructive lung disease causing cor pulmonale
	Acute onset, or an acute exacerbation of cough	An acute respiratory infection precipitating heart failure in a predisposed patient
	Pleuritic pain	Pneumonic illness, or pulmonary embolism, precipitating failure
	Hemoptysis	Pulmonary embolism Mitral stenosis with consequent pulmonary hypertension Eisenmenger's syndrome
Central nervous system	Syncope	An arrhythmia Pulmonary embolism Ischemic heart disease Aortic stenosis Aortic incompetence Idiopathic hypertrophic subaortic stenosis
	Embolic manifestations or transient ischemic attacks	Valvular heart disease An arrhythmia A cardiomyopathy Ischemic heart disease
Genitourinary system	Pregnancy	Precipitation of cardiac failure
Past History		
	Rheumatic fever, known murmur, or "leaking valve"	Valvular heart disease Active carditis Bacterial endocarditis
	Venereal disease	Congenital structure defect Valvular heart disease
	Myocardial infarction Diabetes mellitus Hypercholesterolemia	Ischemic heart disease
	Hypertension	Hypertensive heart disease Ischemic heart disease
	Chronic obstructive lung disease Pulmonary embolic disease	Cor pulmonale

(continued)

Source	Symptom	Potential Significance
Review of the problem list		
	For example:	
	Chronic alcoholism	A cardiomyopathy
	Hemochromatosis	
	Amyloidosis, or	
	A muscular dystrophy	
	Sarcoidosis	A cardiomyopathy
		Cor pulmonale
	Diphtheria	Toxic myocarditis
	Malignant disease	Pulmonary embolism and cor pulmonale
		Irradiation-induced myocarditis
		A drug-induced cardiomyopathy
		Metastatic involvement of the heart or conducting system
		A hyperviscosity syndrome—in a patient with a monoclonal gammopathy
		High output failure due to anemia or fever
	Thyrotoxicosis	High output failure
	Arteriovenous fistulae	
	Paget's disease of bone	
Family History		
	Ischemic heart disease	Ischemic heart disease
	Cerebrovascular disease	
	Peripheral vascular disease	
	Diabetes mellitus	
Life situation		
Occupation	Exposure to dusts	Cor pulmonale
		Pneumoconioses
	High-pressure job	Ischemic heart disease
Medications		
	Digitalis	Toxicity with increasing heart failure
	Radiotherapy	Radiation-induced cardiomyopathy
	Drugs (*e.g.*, Doxorubicin hydrochloride)	Drug-induced cardiomyopathy

(continued)

Source	Symptom	Potential Significance
	Steroids Estrogens	Drug-related fluid retention and overload
	Blood transfusion	Circulatory overload
	Intravenous fluid therapy	
	High sodium chloride intake	
Use of alcohol, cigarettes	Alcohol excesses	Alcoholic cardiomyopathy Beri beri
	Cigarette smoking	Ischemic heart disease
Physical examination		
General appearance	Cyanosis	Cyanotic heart disease—usually congenital defect
		Eisenmenger's syndrome
		Lung disease and cor pulmonale
	Respiratory distress, with use of accessory muscles	Chronic obstructive lung disease and cor pulmonale
	Pursed-lip breathing	
Vital signs		
Blood pressure	Hypertension	Hypertensive heart disease
		Atherosclerotic heart disease
Pulse:		
Rate	Tachycardia	Possibility indicative of high output failure, or a paroxysmal tachycardia, but fairly nonspecific in heart failure
Rhythm	An arrhythmia	See "palpitations," above
Quality	Bounding or full volume	High output failure
	Collapsing	Valvular heart disease—aortic incompetence
	Slow upstroke	Valvular heart disease—aortic stenosis
	A sharp upstroke with twin peaks	Idiopathic hypertrophic subaortic stenosis (a cardiomyopathy)
Temperature	Pyrexia	Bacterial endocarditis; rheumatic fever; an infectious illness, especially pneumonia—precipitating heart failure
		High output failure

(continued)

TABLE 19-2. INFORMATION OF POTENTIAL DIAGNOSTIC VALUE IN DETERMINING THE CAUSE OF CONGESTIVE HEART FAILURE *(Continued)*

Source	Sign	Potential Significance
Respiratory rate	Tachypnea	Failure *per se* Pneumonic illness Pulmonary embolism
The hand	Capillary pulsation	Aortic incompetence
	Warm periphery	High output failure
	Digital artery pulsation	
	Finger clubbing Osler's nodes Splinter hemorrhages	Bacterial endocarditis—as a precipitating factor
Head		
The fundi	Hypertensive retinopathy	Hypertensive heart disease Atherosclerotic heart disease
	Roth spots	Bacterial endocarditis
	Venous engorgement with "boxcar" effect Fundal hemorrhages	Hyperviscosity syndrome
Conjunctivae	Pallor	Anemia—precipitating failure
	Plethora	Congenital cardiac anomaly Primary pulmonary disease
	Petechial hemorrhages	Bacterial endocarditis
Thorax	Signs of chronic obstructive lung disease	Cor pulmonale
	Kyphoscoliosis	
	Signs of consolidation	Precipitation of heart failure by pneumonic illness
Precordium		
Inspection and palpation	Lateral displacement of the apex beat	Cardiac dilatation —resulting from failure —resulting from valvular heart disease Cardiomyopathy (Possibly a noncardiac cause)
	Increased forcefulness of the apex beat	Hypertensive heart disease Aortic stenosis Obstructive cardiomyopathy
	Right ventricular lift	Pulmonary hypertension
	Palpable thrills	Valvular heart disease
	Palpable P2	Pulmonary hypertension
Auscultation		
First heart sound	Increased intensity	Mitral stenosis Hyperkinetic state

(continued)

TABLE 19-2. INFORMATION OF POTENTIAL DIAGNOSTIC VALUE
IN DETERMINING THE CAUSE OF CONGESTIVE HEART FAILURE
(Continued)

Source	Sign	Potential Significance
	Decreased intensity	Cardiac failure, *per se*
		Chronic obstructive lung disease
		Aortic stenosis
Second heart sound	Increased intensity	
	—aortic area	·Systemic hypertension
	—pulmonary area	Pulmonary hypertension
	Reduced intensity	Emphysema (COPD)
		Aortic stenosis
	Abnormal splitting	
	—paradoxical	Left ventricular ejection delay
	—wide	Right ventricular ejection delay
Additional sounds	S4 gallop	Systemic hypertension
		Pulmonary hypertension
		Aortic stenosis
		Subaortic stenosis
		Other cardiomyopathies
		Ischemic heart disease
		Hyperkinetic state
	S3 gallop	Heart failure, *per se*
		Mitral incompetence
	Murmurs	Valvular heart disease
		Structural cardiac abnormalities
		Turbulence due to hyperkinetic blood flow
		Valve ring dilatation resulting from heart failure
Abdomen	Pulsatile hepatomegaly	Tricuspid incompetence
	Splenomegaly	Bacterial endocarditis
		Long-standing heart failure, with cardiac cirrhosis
	Gravid uterus	Precipitation or aggravation of heart failure in pregnancy

On further evaluation of your patient, you establish that she had rheumatic fever at the age of six, manifesting with fever, pain in several joints, and the development of murmurs. She was hospitalized for 6 weeks at the time.

She had a second attack at the age of 9 and was well thereafter until the onset of the dyspnea 2 months ago.

Her pulse rate is 120/min and is strikingly irregular in both rhythm and volume.
Her apex beat is palpable with difficulty, but there is a pronounced "lift" to the left of her sternum.
Pulmonary valve closure is easily palpable.
The first heart sound is increased in intensity.
Initial auscultation is otherwise normal.

What are the more probable reasons for this particular patient's cardiac failure?

- Valvular heart disease is suggested by the history of rheumatic fever and the loud first sound
- An arrhythmia is evident from palpation of the pulse
- Pulmonary hypertension is indicated by the loud and palpable P2 and the right ventricular "lift"

What unifying hypothesis will explain all of these findings?

- Mitral stenosis, with consequent pulmonary hypertension, complicated by atrial fibrillation

Does the absence of the characteristic murmur negate the diagnosis?

No. The characteristic auscultatory findings of mitral stenosis sometimes require very careful and specific auscultation. They may be confined to an area at the apex no bigger than a quarter, and may be audible only with full utilization of all of the maneuvers that might enhance auscultation:

- Exercise
- Posture
- Respiration

Where mitral stenosis is anticipated, auscultation should be undertaken with the "bell," with the patient in the left lateral position, and in full expiration, following a brief period of exercise.

If there is still no audible murmur, does this negate the diagnosis?

No. With so many other indications supporting this diagnosis, laboratory confirmation should be sought:

- Chest radiograph
- ECG
- Echocardiography

Mitral stenosis is confirmed.

It is evident that in the diagnostic approach to this patient, the problem-solving process has progressed through several very definite steps, each requiring formulation, analysis, and investigation. The progression has been:

Swelling of the legs
   ⟶ Generalized edema
      ⟶ Heart failure
         ⟶ Chronic rheumatic heart disease
        ⟶ Mitral stenosis

CHAPTER 20

Ptosis

Drooping of the eyelid is usually asymptomatic. However, it constitutes a useful clinical sign. The presence or absence of ptosis should be consciously and specifically noted in the routine physical examination, especially in those patients in whom it might be anticipated—e.g., patients with malignant disease or diabetes mellitus.

During clinical rounds, you are asked to examine a 45-year-old woman. While inspecting her eyes, you note that she has ptosis on the left side.

What are the likely causes for this finding?

- Neuromuscular disorders
  - A third nerve palsy
  - A sympathetic nerve palsy (Horner's syndrome)
  - Myasthenia gravis
- The possibility of local, regional, or systemic disease that causes drooping of the eyelid because of swelling and edema of the lid should always be remembered.
- A congenital or inherited abnormality is a further consideration.

How might the HISTORY help you to differentiate among these various causes?

The **HISTORY RELEVANT TO THE PROBLEM** might reveal, with regard to

1. Its Onset

- That the patient has "always" been aware of this; or that many in the family have a similar appearance—thus lessening its clinical significance

2. Aggravating or Precipitating Factors

- A recent blow, or other trauma to the eye, or an insect bite—indicative of local pathology, but also possibly indicative of nerve damage

The **REVIEW OF SYSTEMS** might reveal, with regard to

1. The Eye

- Diplopia—suggestive of a third nerve palsy, or of muscular fatigability due to myasthenia gravis

2. The Face

- Dryness of the ipsilateral face, suggestive of Horner's syndrome

3. The Cardiovascular System

- Edema (or swelling) at other sites, suggestive of systemic disease, which would also be the cause of the edema of the eyelid.

How might the physical examination help?

A careful examination of the head should provide diagnostically useful information. With regard to

1. The Eyelids

- Swelling and/or discoloration of the lid would obviously suggest local pathology—possibly a systemic illness associated with edema, and possibly more serious local pathology involving the cavernous sinus or nerves.
- The ability to retract the lid with voluntary effort would favor Horner's syndrome. Failure of such voluntary retraction would strongly favor a third nerve palsy.

2. The Pupils

- Inequality of pupil size would be of tremendous diagnostic value:

○ A constricted pupil on the ipsilateral side would be virtually diagnostic of Horner's syndrome. A widely dilated pupil on that side would indicate a third nerve palsy.

3. The Pupillary Reflexes

- Failure of the pupil to dilate with diminished light would suggest Horner's syndrome;
- Loss of the pupillary reflex to light and accommodation on the affected side, with retention of the consensual light reflex, would strongly favor a third nerve palsy.

4. The Eye Movements, and Position of the Eyes

- Resting lateral deviation of the affected eye would indicate a third nerve palsy; so would paralysis or paresis of inward, downward, and upward gaze of the affected eye.

MYASTHENIA GRAVIS

Under what circumstances would you consider the possibility of myasthenia gravis more seriously?

- If the history or physical examination to this point had failed to confirm a third nerve palsy, Horner's syndrome, edema, or other local pathology of the eyelid
- If both lids were involved
- If the sign worsened with sustained effort
- If the oculomotor signs fluctuated

How might the HISTORY further the suspicion of myasthenia gravis?

The **HISTORY RELEVANT TO THE PROBLEM** might reveal:

- The occurrence of diplopia and ptosis toward the end of the day, with improvement after a night's rest

The **SYSTEMS REVIEW** might reveal, with regard to

1. Her General Health

- Increasing fatigability, especially evident at the end of the day

2. The Gastrointestinal System

- Difficulty chewing and difficulty in swallowing, possibly with nasal regurgitation, with progression of these symptoms over the course of a meal

2. The Nervous System

- Slurring of speech, worsening with effort

3. The Locomotor System

- Increasing, but reversible, muscle fatigability—especially evident at the end of the day, and/or with sustained effort, *e.g.*, brushing teeth, climbing stairs, combing hair, etc.

The **PROBLEM LIST** or **PAST HISTORY** might reveal the presence of other disorders known to be associated with myasthenia gravis, increasing its probability—*e.g.*

- Rheumatoid arthritis
- Sjögren's syndrome
- Thyrotoxicosis
- A malignancy
- A thymoma
- Polymyositis
- A congenital myopathy

The **FAMILY HISTORY** might reveal an established diagnosis of myasthenia gravis in other family members.

How might the PHYSICAL EXAMINATION help in pursuing this diagnosis?

The following signs might be discovered through examination of the

1. Head and Neck

- Inability to *sustain* the muscular effort necessary for
  - Upward gaze
  - Tight closure of the eyes
  - Smiling
  - Counting up to 100, or speaking at length—so that slurring of speech occurs

2. Nervous System

- Inability to sustain muscular effort, especially of proximal muscle groups

THIRD NERVE PALSY

What features would enable you to diagnose a third nerve palsy?

A history of

- Diplopia

Physical findings:

- Lateral deviation of the affected eye
- An inability to deviate the eye fully inward, upward, or downward
- A fixed, dilated pupil

If a third nerve palsy were to be confirmed on the basis of these features, how should you proceed?

The question to be posed will change from:

- "Why does this patient have ptosis?"

to:

- "Why does this patient have a third nerve palsy?"

At what anatomical sites might the third nerve be damaged?

- In the midbrain
- At the base of the brain in the subarachnoid space
- In the cavernous sinus
- In the superior orbital fissure
- Within the orbit

What are the likely causes for damage at these various sites?

- Midbrain
  ○ Cerebrovascular disease

- ○ Tumor
- • Base of brain
  - ○ Meningitis
  - ○ Berry aneurysm
  - ○ Temporal lobe herniation
  - ○ Malignant disease
- • Cavernous sinus
  - ○ Thrombosis
  - ○ Arteriovenous fistula
- • Superior orbital fissure
  - ○ Trauma
  - ○ Tumor
- • Orbit
  - ○ Cellulitis/abscess
  - ○ Tumor
- • Vasculitis
  - ○ Diabetes mellitus
- • Idiopathic—cause and site unknown

How might the HISTORY and PHYSICAL EXAMINATION assist you in establishing the anatomical location and/or cause of this nerve palsy?

Symptoms and signs that might have diagnostic value are listed in Table 20-1.

TABLE 20-1.   SYMPTOMS AND SIGNS OF POTENTIAL DIAGNOSTIC SIGNIFICANCE IN A PATIENT WITH A THIRD NERVE PALSY

Source	Symptom	Potential Significance
Review of Systems		
General Health	Fever	Meningitis
		Cavernous sinus thrombosis
	Weight loss	Diabetes mellitus
		Malignant disease with metastases
ENT	Pain in, or discharge from the ear; deafness	Disease of the ear, mastoids, nose, or paranasal sinuses that may have presaged the development of
	A nasal discharge, an intranasal furuncle, or sinus pain	Meningitis Cavernous or paranasal sinus thrombosis
		(A third nerve palsy is usually a late sign).

(continued)

TABLE 20-1. SYMPTOMS AND SIGNS OF POTENTIAL DIAGNOSTIC SIGNIFICANCE IN A PATIENT WITH A THIRD NERVE PALSY *(Continued)*

Source	Symptom	Potential Significance
Skin	Facial furuncle	Cavernous sinus thrombosis
Central nervous system	Headache	Diabetes mellitus
		Berry aneurysm
		Meningitis
		Cavernous sinus thrombosis
		Intracranial mass lesion
	Weakness, paralysis, tremor, or hemi-anesthesia of the contralateral limbs	Midbrain pathology Cerebrovascular disease Tumor Supratentorial mass lesion with impending herniation
	Impaired sensation over the ipsilateral face	Simultaneous fifth cranial nerve involvement—suggestive of cavernous sinus disease
Respiratory system	Cough, hemoptysis chest pain, dyspnea, or wheezing	Possible bronchogenic malignancy with intracranial metastases
Genitourinary system	Polyuria	Diabetes mellitus
Past History or Review of Problem List	Trauma—accidental or surgical—to the head	Direct damage to the nerve at the base of the brain, or in the orbit
		Intracranial hemorrhage and incipient transtentorial herniation of the uncus
	Infection	
	Mastoiditis	Meningitis
	Sinusitis	Brain abscess
	Tuberculosis	Tuberculous meningitis
	Malignant disease	An ipsilateral supratentorial metastasis with incipient herniation
		Very rarely—metastatic involvement of the third nerve nucleus or its fibers
		Opportunistic meningeal infection
		Side effect of chemotherapy, especially vincristine
	Subarachnoid hemorrhage	Posterior communicating artery aneurysm

(continued)

226

TABLE 20-1. SYMPTOMS AND SIGNS OF POTENTIAL DIAGNOSTIC
SIGNIFICANCE IN A PATIENT WITH A THIRD NERVE PALSY
(Continued)

Source	Symptom	Potential Significance
	Atherosclerotic disease (*e.g.*, ischemic heart disease, transient ischemic attacks, strokes, peripheral vascular disease)	Cerebrovascular accident with involvement of midbrain structures
	Diabetes mellitus	Diabetic neuropathy
		Cerebrovascular disease
Family History	Diabetes	Diabetic neuropathy
		Cerebrovascular disease
Physical Examination		
General appearance	Acutely ill	Meningitis
		Cavernous sinus thrombosis
Vital signs	Pyrexia	Meningitis
		Cavernous sinus thrombosis
	Hypertension	Atherosclerotic cerebrovascular disease
		Ruptured berry aneurysm
		Large intracranial bleed
Mental status	Altered level of consciousness	Meningeal involvement by infection or tumor
		An intracranial mass lesion
		Midbrain involvement by vascular disease or tumor
Head		Ruptured berry aneurysm
Scalp	Evidence of trauma	Damage to nerve
		Meningitis
		Mass lesion
Eye	Edema of the eyelid	Cavernous sinus thrombosis
	Xanthelasmata	Diabetic neuropathy
	Sparing of the pupil	Diabetic neuropathy
	Additional paralysis of fourth and sixth ipsilateral cranial nerves	Meningeal disease
		Cavernous sinus thrombosis or aneurysm
		Superior orbital fissure disease
	Ipsilateral impairment of visual acuity	Tumor at orbital apex
		Cavernous sinus thrombosis

(continued)

TABLE 20-1. SYMPTOMS AND SIGNS OF POTENTIAL DIAGNOSTIC SIGNIFICANCE IN A PATIENT WITH A THIRD NERVE PALSY *(Continued)*

Source	Symptom	Potential Significance
	Exophthalmos	Intraorbital tumor
		Cavernous sinus thrombosis
	Chemosis	Cavernous sinus thrombosis
Fundus	Papilledema	Meningitis
		Intracranial mass lesion
		Cavernous sinus thrombosis
	Optic atrophy	Orbital disease
	Subhyaloid hemorrhage	Subarchnoid hemorrhage from ruptured berry aneurysm
	Diabetic retinopathy	Diabetic neuropathy
	Hypertensive retinopathy	See "Hypertension," above
Ear	Discharge	Meningitis
	Change in drum	Cavernous sinus thrombosis
	Cholesteatoma	Cerebral abscess
Face	Edema of unilateral face	Cavernous sinus disease
	Loss of sensation over first and second divisions of the fifth cranial nerve	
Neck	Neck stiffness	Meningeal involvement: infection,
	Brudzinski's sign	hemorrhage, tumor
	Lymphadenopathy especially left supraclavicular area	Malignant disease with possible intracranial metastases
Chest	Abnormalities that could be compatible with carcinoma of the lung	Intracranial metastases
Breast	Mastectomy scar	Possible intracranial metastases
	Breast lump	
Extremities	Involuntary movements	Midbrain pathology
		Intracranial mass lesion
	Increased tone, paresis, or paralysis	Possibly meningitis
	Hyperreflexia	
	Extensor plantar response	
	Hemianesthesia	
	Kernig's sign	Meningeal irritation by infection, tumor or hemorrhage

During the course of the interview, you learn that the patient had been quite well until about a week ago. She then developed a severe pain in the area of her left eye and forehead, which was followed in 2 days by the development of ptosis and diplopia. There are no other significant symptoms.

What disorders would this history particularly suggest?

- A berry aneurysm of the posterior communicating artery
- Diabetes mellitus

Less likely, but possible considerations would also include:

- Cavernous sinus thrombosis
- Meningitis
- An intracranial mass lesion

What clinical features would support a diagnosis of:

1. A Berry Aneurysm?

In the

- Fundus
  - Subhyaloid hemorrhages
- Neck
  - Neck stiffness
  - Brudzinski's sign
- Extremities
  - Kernig's sign

2. Diabetes Mellitus?

- Sparing of the pupil would very much support this diagnosis.
- The symptoms and signs that should be considered are discussed at length in the chapter on "Polyuria."

3. Cavernous Sinus Thrombosis?

With regard to

- General appearance
  - A toxic, acutely ill appearance
- Vital signs
  - Pyrexia

- Eyes
  - Edema of the forehead, eyelid, base of nose
  - Proptosis
  - Hyperesthesia of the forehead
  - Accompanying paralysis of the fourth and sixth cranial nerves
  - Chemosis
  - Retinal changes: retinal vein engorgement, retinal hemorrhages, papilledema

4. Meningitis?

With regard to

- General appearance
  - An acutely ill, toxic appearance
- Vital signs
  - Pyrexia
- Fundi
  - Papilledema
- Neck
  - Neck stiffness
  - Brudzinski's sign
- Extremities
  - Kernig's sign

5. A Mass Lesion?

With regard to

- Fundi
  - Papilledema
- Cranial nerves and extremities
  - Lateralizing signs

What investigations are indicated to test your specific diagnostic suspicions?

- A radiograph of the skull
- A CAT scan of the head
- Blood glucose concentration assays
- Perhaps carotid arteriography

- A lumbar puncture—obviously important, but to be undertaken with caution and with the guidance of a neurologist, if there is any suspicion of raised intracranial pressure.

HORNER'S SYNDROME

What constellation of findings would enable you to diagnose Horner's syndrome?

- A history of
  - Dryness of the affected cheek
- Physical signs:
  - Mild ptosis
  - A contracted pupil
  - Dryness of the ipsilateral face
  - (Possibly enophthalmos)

What are the likely causes of a Horner's syndrome?

- Involvement of the cervical sympathetic chain by
  - Malignant disease—especially carcinoma of the lung or a lymphoma
  - Trauma—as part of a birth injury or other major injury involving the neck, or in the course of carotid arteriography or neck surgery
- Damage to the sympathetic fibers in the C8, T1, roots
  - Usually on a traumatic or a malignant basis
- Damage to the cervical spinal cord, with involvement of the intermediolateral columns by cervical spondylitis, or tumor
- Brainstem involvement of the sympathetic fibers, particularly by vascular disease and tumor
- Heterochromia iridis—a common benign disorder combining Horner's syndrome and a depigmented iris

How might you attempt to differentiate among these disorders?

The **SYSTEMS REVIEW** might reveal, with regard to

1. The Locomotor System

- A history of neck pain with radiation into the hand
- Paresthesias in the hand

These are symptoms very suggestive of *cervical cord* or C8 and T1 *root involvement.*

2. The Nervous System

- "Brainstem" symptoms
  - ○ Vertigo, nausea, and vomiting
  - ○ Dysarthria
  - ○ Dysphasia
  - ○ Loss of balance
  - ○ Impaired coordination
- Weakness of the legs—suggestive of *cervical cord* or *brainstem involvement*

A **REVIEW OF THE PAST HISTORY** or **PROBLEM LIST** might reveal evidence of

- Birth injury, or other major injury to the neck
- Recent carotid arteriography or neck surgery
- Known cervical spondylitis
- Known malignant disease

—all with localizing significance, as discussed above.

PHYSICAL EXAMINATION might reveal

1. In the Hand

- Wasting of the small muscles
- A characteristic claw-hand deformity
- Paralysis of the intrinsic muscles of the hand, and flexors of the wrist and fingers
- Sensory loss over the ulnar border of the hand and inner surface of the forearm

—all suggestive of C8 and T1 *root involvement.*

2. In the Head

- Depigmentation of the iris—suggestive of heterochromia iridis

- "Brainstem" signs of
  - ○ Nystagmus
  - ○ Palatal paralysis
  - ○ Loss of palatal reflexes
  - ○ Wasting and fasciculation of the tongue
  - ○ Weakness of the trapezius and sternomastoid muscles

3. In the Neck

- Limitation of neck movement—suggestive of *cervical root* or *cervical cord* pathology
- Lymphadenopathy or other neck pathology—suggestive of *sympathetic chain* involvement

4. In the Lower Limbs

- Long-tract sensory and motor signs—suggestive of *brainstem* or *cervical cord* disease

Once the site of the lesion has been established, it is then necessary to determine the cause.

In the patient with an isolated Horner's syndrome of recent onset, the possibility of occult malignant disease requires careful consideration (see Chap. 2).

Bedside medicine can be exhilirating, and the diagnostic process satisfying and exciting. Much of it is concerned with asking the appropriate questions at the right time, and with following an orderly routine in pursuing and interpreting the answers (although the value of an occasional flash of inspiration is not to be gainsaid).

Clinical reasoning begins immediately upon contact with a patient. As information is gathered, so diagnostic hypotheses are generated, tested, and refined.

The intent of this book has been to stress the role of the orderly history and physical examination in this process—not as a mindless, obsessive-compulsive exercise, but rather as a means to an end. The goal is not to gather routine information, but, on the contrary, to seek, in a careful, conscious, and orderly fashion, specific evidence upon which to base an individualized and well-reasoned differential diagnosis.

SUGGESTED READING

This book was not written in isolation, and it is not intended that it be read thus. The following books were, and should be, liberally consulted:

BOOKS ON PHYSICAL DIAGNOSIS

Bouchier IAD, Morris JS: Clinical Skills. Philadelphia, W.B. Saunders, 1976

De Gowin EL, De Gowin RL: Bedside Diagnostic Examination, 3rd ed. New York, MacMillan, 1976

Hunter D, Bomford RR: Hutchison's Clinical Methods. London, Cassell, 1956

Judge RD, Zuidema GD (eds): Physical Diagnosis, 3rd ed. Boston, Little, Brown, 1974

MacBryde CM, Blacklow RS (eds): Signs and Symptoms, 5th ed. Philadelphia, J.B. Lippincott, 1970

MacLeod J (ed): Clinical Examination, 4th ed. Edinburgh and London, Churchill Livingstone, 1976

Morgan WL, Engel GL: The Clinical Approach to the Patient. Philadelphia, W.B. Saunders, 1969

Reller LB, Sahn SA, Schrier RW (eds): Clinical Internal Medicine. Boston, Little, Brown, 1979

Walker HK, Hall WD, Hirst JW (eds): Clinical Methods. Boston, Butterworth, 1976

TEXTBOOKS OF MEDICINE

Beeson PB, McDermott W: Cecil-Loeb Textbook of Medicine, 15th ed. Philadelphia, W.B. Saunders, 1979 (in press)

Harvey AM, Bordley J: Differential Diagnosis, 3rd ed. Philadelphia, W.B. Saunders, 1979 (in press)

Harvey AM, Johns RJ, Owens AH, Ross RS: The Principles and Practice of Medicine, 19th ed. New York, Appleton-Century-Crofts, 1976

MacLeod J. (ed): Davidson's Principles and Practice of Medicine, 11th ed. Edinburgh, London, New York, Churchill Livingstone, 1975

Thorn GW, Adams RD, Braunwald E, Isselbacher KJ, Petersdorf RG (eds): Harrison's Principles of Internal Medicine, 8th ed. New York, McGraw-Hill, 1977

INDEX

Numerals followed by a t indicate a table.

Acute dyspnea,
  abdominal signs and, 38
  airway obstruction and, 33, 36
  appearance of patient and, 35
  blood analysis and, 34
  cardiovascular signs and, 34
  causes of, 30–31
  central nervous system signs and, 34
  chest signs and, 32–33, 36–39, 52
  extremity symptoms and, 38
  family history and, 35
  general health of patient with, 33
  head symptoms and, 36
  history of patient with, 33, 35
  infection and, 39
  laboratory tests and, 34, 39
  leukemic patient with, 30–39
  neck symptoms and, 36
  physical examination and, 32–34, 35–39
  precordial signs and, 37–38
  pulmonary embolism and, 39
  respiratory signs and, 34
  sputum analysis, 35
  tension pneumothorax and, 32, 36–37
  thoracic signs and, 32–33, 36–37
  vital signs and, 35

Bleeders. *See* Easy bruising
Bruising. *See* Easy bruising

Cardiac failure. *See* Heart failure
Central chest pain,
  abdominal signs and, 54, 57
  alcohol consumption and, 55
  cardiovascular signs and, 52
  causes of, 45, 50, 54–55
  central nervous system symptoms and, 53
  chest examination and, 56
  cigarette smoking and, 48
  clubbing of the fingers and, 150–151
  cord compression and, 53–57
  description of 47, 50, 55
  diabetes mellitus and, 86t
  dissecting aneurysms and, 50–51
  dyspnea and, 40–41
  extremity symptoms and, 49, 53–55
  family history and, 48
  gastrointestinal signs and, 55–56
  general appearance of patient with, 48, 50, 52
  hand symptoms and, 51
  head symptoms and, 49, 51–52
  history of patient and, 46–48, 50, 52–54
  hoarseness and, 27
  hypotension and, 142
  laboratory studies and, 46, 49–51, 53–54, 57
  life situation and, 48, 56
  lung signs and, 49
  mental status and, 50
  neck symptoms and, 49, 51–52
  peripheral edema and, 206
  physical examination of patient with, 46, 48–54, 56–57
  precordial signs and, 49, 51, 53
  ptosis and, 266t
  pulmonary embolism and, 51–53
  rectal examination and, 54
  respiratory signs and, 52
  root compression and, 53–57
  splenomegaly and, 194
  thoracic signs and, 51

235

Central chest pain, *(continued)*
  vital signs and, 49–50, 52
  vomiting and, 64t
Chest, dullness to percussion of the.
  See Dullness to percussion of
    the chest
Chest pain, central. *See* Central chest
  pain
Clinical findings, evaluation of, 2–6
Clubbing of the fingers,
  abdominal symptoms and, 154–155
  alcohol consumption and, 152
  cardiovascular signs and, 150
  case of a man with, 149, 150, 156
  causes of, 149–150, 156
  clinical significance of, 149
  drug addiction and, 152
  extremity signs and, 154
  family history and, 152
  gastrointestinal symptoms and, 151
  general appearance of patient with,
    154
  general health of patient with, 150
  genitourinary symptoms and, 151
  hand symptoms and, 153–154
  head symptoms and, 153, 157
  heart failure and, 216
  history of patient with, 150–152
  jaundice and, 183
  laboratory studies and, 154
  life situation and, 152
  lung symptoms and, 155
  musculoskeletal symptoms and, 151
  neck symptoms and, 153, 156
  neurologic signs and, 154
  occupational history and, 152
  physical examination of patient
    with, 153–156
  pleural effusion and, 171
  precordial symptoms and, 153, 155
  rectal signs and, 156
  respiratory symptoms and, 151
  skin symptoms and, 151, 153
  tobacco use and, 152
  vital signs and, 153–154
  weight loss and, 21, 19t

Dullness to percussion of the chest,
  atelectasis as cause of, 162
  auscultation and, 161, 162
  causes of, 157, 161
  chest examination and, 157–162

consolidation as cause of, 161
  clubbing of the fingers and, 156
  dyspnea and, 36–37, 42t
  laboratory studies and, 160–161
  pleural fluid as cause of, 161–162
Dyspnea,
  See also Acute dyspnea, Dyspnea on
    exertion
  chest pain and, 46–47, 52
  clubbing of the fingers and, 150–151
  heart failure and, 217t
  hypotension and, 142
  pleural effusion and, 175, 167t
  ptosis and, 226t
  splenomegaly and, 194
  vomiting and, 64t
  weight loss and, 21
Dyspnea on exertion,
  abdominal signs and, 42t
  alcohol consumption and, 44
  breast cancer and, 39–40, 43–44,
    41t, 42t
  cardiovascular signs and, 40, 43
  causes of, 40
  cigarette use and, 44
  extremity symptoms and, 43t
  family history and, 43
  general appearance of patient with,
    41t
  head signs and, 41t
  history of patient with, 40, 43–44
  hoarseness and, 27
  laboratory studies and, 44
  life situation and, 43–44
  medication history and, 44
  peripheral edema and, 206, 209
  physical examination of patient
    with, 32–38, 40–41, 43–44, 41t,
    42t, 43t
  pleural fluid and, 166
  precordial signs and, 42t
  neck signs and, 41t
  radiotherapeutic history of patient
    with, 44
  respiratory symptoms and, 43
  thoracic symptoms and, 41t
  vital signs and, 41t

Easy bruising,
  abdominal symptoms and, 106
  case histories of patients showing,
    108–111

Easy bruising, *(continued)*
  causes of, 107, 109–110, 112
  clinical features of, 102–103
  ear symptoms and, 103
  eye symptoms and, 103, 106
  family history and, 103, 105, 107,
    109–111
  gastrointestinal symptoms and, 104
  genitourinary symptoms, 104
  hand symptoms and, 106
  history of patient with, 103–104,
    110
  jaundice and, 83
  laboratory studies and, 106–107,
    111–112
  mechanisms of, 107
  medication history and, 105
  mouth symptoms and, 106
  musculoskeletal signs and, 105
  nasal symptoms and, 103
  physical examination and, 105–106
  polyuria and, 77t
  postoperative patients with, 105
  respiratory symptoms and, 104
  skin symptoms and, 104–105
  throat symptoms and, 103

Headache(s),
  abdominal symptoms and, 119
  acute, 113–119
  cancer patient with, 124
  cases of women with, 113, 120
  causes of, 114–115, 118, 120
  central nervous system symptoms
    and, 114–115, 123
  characteristics of, 120–122
  diabetes mellitus and, 85t
  ear symptoms and, 117–118, 123
  extremity symptoms and, 117, 119,
    125
  eye symptoms and, 115–118, 123
  family history and, 124
  gastrointestinal symptoms and, 118
  general appearance of patient with,
    116, 119
  general health of patient with, 114,
    118, 123
  genitourinary symptoms and, 119
  head symptoms and, 116, 119, 125
  history of patient with, 114–115,
    120, 123–124
  hypertension and, 129, 131–132

  laboratory investigations and, 117,
    125
  life situation and, 115–116
  mental status and, 116, 119, 125
  mouth symptoms and, 117
  musculoskeletal symptoms and, 119,
    123
  neck symptoms and, 117, 119, 125
  nasal symptoms and, 118, 123
  physical examination and, 114,
    116–119
  polyuria and, 77t
  precordial symptoms and, 125
  ptosis and, 226t
  skin symptoms and, 119
  recurrent, 120–125
  respiratory symptons and, 118
  skin symptoms and, 119,
  throat symptoms and, 118, 123
  trauma preceding, 124
  vital signs and, 116, 119, 125
  vomiting and, 69, 63t
  weight loss and, 16
Heart failure,
  abdominal signs and, 217t
  alcohol consumption and, 215t
  anatomical basis of, 211
  cardiovascular symptoms and, 212t
  case of woman with, 217–219
  causes of, 211
  central nervous system symptoms
    and, 213t
  chest pain and, 45–46
  cigarette smoking and, 215t
  clinical significance of, 126–129
  diagnostic approach to, 212, 213t,
    214t, 215t, 216t, 217t
  dyspnea and, 43–44, 41t, 42t
  eye symptoms and, 130
  family history and, 214t
  first heart sound in, 216t
  general appearance of patient with,
    215t
  genitourinary symptoms and, 213t
  hand symptoms and, 216t
  head symptoms and, 216t
  heart murmur and, 218
  heart signs and, 216t, 217t
  history of patient with, 213t, 214t
  hypertension and, 131, 131t, 217t
  medication history and, 214t, 215t
  occupational history and, 214t
  peripheral edema and, 205–206,
    209–210, 208t

Heart failure, *(continued)*
  physical examination of patient
    with, 212t, 213t, 215t, 216t,
    217t
  pleural effusion and, 171–172
  precordial signs and, 216t
  respiratory symptoms and, 213t
  second heart sound in, 217t
  thoracic signs and, 216t
  vital signs and, 215t
  vomiting and, 60
Hoarseness,
  cardiovascular symptoms and, 27, 29
  causes of, 23–24
  clinical significance of, 23
  clubbing of the fingers and, 151
  gastrointestinal symptoms and, 27
  general appearance of patient with,
    26, 28
  general health of patient with, 25,
    27
  genitourinary symptoms and, 27
  head symptoms and, 26, 28
  history of patient with, 25, 27–28
  laryngoscopic examination of
    patient with, 29
  life situation and, 25–26
  mental status and, 28
  musculoskeletal symptoms and, 27
  myxedema and, 26–29
  neck symptoms and, 26, 28–29
  neurologic symptoms and, 24, 27, 29
  physical examination of patient
    with, 26–29
  pleural effusion and, 171
  respiratory symptoms and, 25
  skin symptoms and, 27, 29
  tomographic examination of patient
    with, 29
  vital signs and, 28
Hypertension,
  abdominal signs and, 133t, 137t
  cardiovascular symptoms and,
    130–131
  causes of, 134–137
  central nervous system symptoms
    and, 130–132
  cerebrovascular disease and, 129
  chest pain and, 49
  clinical significance of, 133
  determination of, 126–127
  diabetes mellitus and, 86t
  diagnostic factors in patient with,
    126

drug history and, 124, 136
effects of, 129–134
extremity signs and, 134t, 137t
eye symptoms and, 133t
facial symptoms and, 133t
family history and, 136
finger clubbing and, 216
food history and, 136
general appearance of patient with,
  133t, 137t
genitourinary symptoms and, 132,
  135
head symptoms and, 133, 137t
headache and, 115, 120, 124
heart failure and, 129, 211, 213t
history of patient with, 130, 135
laboratory studies and, 134, 136–
  139
lung signs and, 133t
mental status and, 133t
neck signs and, 133t, 137t
nervous system symptoms and, 134t
peripheral edema and, 208t
physical examination of patient
  with, 125, 133
pleural effusion and, 171
precordial signs and, 133t
prognostic factors for, 126
renal diseases and, 130
thoracic signs and, 137t
vital signs and, 133t, 137t
Hypotension,
  abdominal signs and, 144–145
  cardiovascular symptoms and, 142
  case of a woman with breast cancer
    and, 138–147
  causes of, 138–141, 145–146
  chest pain and, 46, 49, 52
  clinical significance of, 138, 147
  dehydration and, 81
  diabetes mellitus and, 86t
  drug history and, 143
  effects of, 147–148
  extremity symptoms and, 145
  gastrointestinal symptoms and, 145
  general health of patient with,
    142–143
  head symptoms and, 144
  history of patient with, 142–143,
    146
  laboratory studies and, 145–147
  neck symptoms and, 144
  physical examination of patient
    with, 143–146

Hypotension, *(continued)*
  pleural effusion and, 170
  precordial symptoms and, 144
  rectal signs and, 145
  respiratory symptoms and, 142
  skin symptoms and, 145
  thoracic symptoms and, 144
  vital signs and, 143
  vomiting and, 70, 72–73

Interviewing the patient,
  general procedure for, 2–6

Jaundice,
  abdominal signs and, 184
  alcohol consumption and, 182
  bilirubin levels in serum and, 177
  case of woman with, 178, 185–186
  causes of, 177–179, 185
  characteristics of, 176–177
  chest pain and, 56
  clinical significance of, 177
  clubbing of the fingers and, 151, 155
  confirmation of, 177
  discoloration of the skin and, 176
  drug addiction and, 182
  extremity signs and, 184
  gastrointestinal symptoms and, 180
  general appearance of patient with,
    183
  general health of patient with, 180
  hand symptoms and, 183
  head symptoms and, 183
  hepatoxin exposure and, 182
  history of patient with, 176, 178–
    182, 185
  hobbies of patient with, 182
  hyperbilirubinemia and, 186
  laboratory studies and, 186
  life situation and, 181–182
  medication history and, 182
  mental status and, 183
  neck symptoms and, 183
  occupational history and, 181–182
  peripheral edema and, 206, 208t
  personal problems and, 182
  physical examination of patient
    with, 176, 179, 183–185
  pleural effusion and, 171
  scrotal signs and, 184

skin symptoms and, 176–177, 181,
    183–184
  splenomegaly and, 191
  thoracic signs and, 184
  vital signs and, 183
  vomiting and, 60, 63t
  weight loss and, 14
Joint pain,
  abdominal signs and, 94, 97
  acute arthritis causing, 98–101
  aspiration of the joint in patient
    with, 101
  back symptoms and, 101
  cardiovascular signs and, 91, 96
  case of man with, 98
  case of woman with, 88
  causes of, 88, 98
  chest symptoms and, 94
  drug history and, 92, 100
  ear symptoms and, 96–97
  extremity symptoms and, 94, 96–97,
    101
  eye symptoms and, 92
  family history and, 92, 100
  gastrointestinal signs and, 91, 99
  general appearance of patient and,
    93, 100
  general health of patient and, 90, 99
  genitourinary symptoms and, 99,
    101
  hair loss and, 91
  head symptoms and, 93, 101
  heart failure and, 217t
  hemopoietic symptoms and, 96
  history of patient with, 100
  inflammatory polyarthritis causing,
    90–95
  laboratory studies and, 94, 97, 101
  life situation and, 92, 100
  locomotor system symptoms and, 91,
    99
  mental status and, 92
  nail symptoms and, 91, 93
  nasal symptoms and, 96, 98
  neck symptoms and, 93, 101
  nervous system symptoms and, 92,
    96
  osteoarthritis and, 89–90
  physical examination of patient
    with, 89–90, 92–94, 97, 100–
    101
  pleural effusion and, 167t
  polyarthritis causing, 89, 95
  precordial signs and, 94

Joint pain, *(continued)*
  respiratory signs and, 91
  rheumatoid arthritis causing,
    90–101
  skin symptoms and, 90–91, 93, 99
  splenomegaly and, 199
  systemic lupus erythematosus as
    cause of, 90–94
  throat symptoms and, 96, 99
  vital signs and, 93, 101
  weight loss and, 16

Percussion of the chest, dullness to.
    See Dullness to percussion of
    the chest
Peripheral edema,
  abdominal signs and, 209, 208t
  cardiovascular symptoms and, 206
  case of a patient with, 205–210
  chest symptoms and, 206
  clubbing of the fingers and, 150
  diabetes mellitus and, 86t
  distribution of, 204
  dyspnea and, 43t
  genitourinary signs and, 206
  hand symptoms and, 206
  head symptoms and, 208t
  heart failure and, 219
  history of patient with, 205–207
  hypertension and, 134t
  inflammatory features associated
    with, 204–20
  laboratory studies and, 209
  life situation and, 207
  local versus systemic, 204
  lung signs and, 209
  medication history and, 207
  mental status and, 208t
  neck symptoms and, 209, 208t
  physical examination of patient
    with, 207, 209, 210, 208t
  pleural effusion and, 173
  precordial signs and, 209, 208t
  ptosis and, 221
  systemic versus local, 204
  vital signs and, 209, 208t
Pleural effusion,
  abdominal signs and, 160, 172–173
  alcohol consumption and, 170, 169t
  axillary hair and, 172
  axillary lymph nodes and, 172
  breast signs and, 172

cardiovascular symptoms and, 167t
case of man with, 165–166, 169
causes of, 164, 169–170
chest symptoms and, 51, 172
cigarette smoking and, 169t
differential diagnosis of, major
  factors in, 165
dullness to percussion of the chest
  and, 159–161
dyspnea and, 31, 33–34, 37, 40, 43,
  41t
effects of, 175
extremity signs and, 173
family history and, 168t
gastrointestinal symptoms and, 167t
general appearance of patient with,
  170
general health of patient with, 166t
hand symptoms and, 171
head symptoms and, 171
history of patient and, 166, 168, 170,
  166t, 167t, 168t, 169t
laboratory tests and, 173–174
life situation and, 168t
medication history and, 169t
musculoskeletal symptoms and, 167t
nature of, 163–164
neck symptoms and, 171
pelvic signs in woman with, 173
peripheral edema and, 205, 208t
physical examination of patient
  with, 170–173
precordial signs and, 172
rectal signs and, 172–173
respiratory signs and, 167t
scrotal symptoms and, 172–173
skin symptoms and, 167, 170
thoracic signs and, 171–172
vital signs and, 170–171
Polyuria,
  alcohol consumption and, 83, 78t
  cardiovascular symptoms and, 84,
    86t
  case of woman with, 74–75, 82
  causes of, 75–76
  central nervous system symptoms
    and, 85t
  clinical significance of, 75
  confirmation of, 74
  definition of, 74
  dehydration and, 81–82
  diabetes mellitus and, 79–85, 85t,
    86t, 87t
  extremity symptoms and, 81

Polyuria, *(continued)*
  eye symptoms and, 75, 85t
  family history and, 83–84, 78t
  gastrointestinal symptoms and, 83,
    77t, 86t
  general appearance of patient with,
    80, 84
  genitourinary symptoms and, 79,
    77t, 86t, 87t
  hand symptoms and, 86t
  head symptoms and, 80, 82, 84, 86t
  history of patient with, 76, 83, 77t,
    85t, 86t, 87t
  hypertension and, 132, 136
  laboratory tests and, 79–82, 87t
  life situation and, 78t
  manifestations of, 74
  medication history and, 83, 78t
  mental status and, 80, 84, 86t
  neck symptoms and, 84
  nervous system symptoms and, 77t,
    87t
  physical examination of patient
    with, 79–82, 84, 85t, 86t, 87t
  precordial signs and, 81
  psychological status and, 77t
  ptosis and, 229, 226t
  skin symptoms and, 79–80, 82, 84,
    77t, 86t, 87t
  vital signs and, 80–81, 84, 86t
  vomiting and, 63t
Ptosis,
  breast symptoms and, 228t
  cardiovascular symptoms and, 221
  case of woman with, 220, 229
  causes of, 220–221, 224–225, 231
  central nervous system symptoms
    and, 226t
  chest symptoms and, 228t
  ear symptoms and, 225t, 228t
  extremity signs and, 229–230, 233,
    228t
  eye symptoms and, 221–222, 229–
    230, 227t, 228t
  eyelid symptoms and, 220–221, 227t
  facial symptoms and, 221, 228t
  family history and, 223, 227t
  fundus symptoms and, 229–230,
    228t
  gastrointestinal symptoms and, 223
  general appearance of patient with,
    229–230, 227t
  general health of patient with, 222,
    225t

genitourinary symptoms and, 226t
hand symptoms and, 232
head symptoms and, 223, 229–230,
  232–233, 227t
Horner's syndrome and, 232–233
laboratory studies and, 230–231
locomotor system symptoms and,
  232
mental status and, 227t
myasthenia gravis as cause of,
  222–224
neck symptoms and, 223, 229–230,
  233, 228t
nasal symptoms and, 225t
nervous system symptoms and,
  223–224, 230, 232
physical examination of patient
  with, 221–224, 231–233, 225t,
  226t, 227t, 228t
pupillary signs and, 221–222
respiratory symptoms and, 226t
skin symptoms and, 226t
third nerve palsy as cause of, 224–
  225, 229, 225t, 226t, 227t, 228t
vital signs and, 229–230, 227t

Splenomegaly,
  abdominal signs and, 191, 202, 196t,
    197t
  axillary signs and, 191, 201, 196t
  blood test and, 189
  cardiovascular signs and, 194, 199
  case of a chronically ill patient with,
    192–195, 197, 195t, 196t, 197t
  case of a patient with, 189–192
  case of an acutely ill patient with,
    197–203
  causes of, 189–190, 192–193, 198
  central nervous system symptoms
    and, 92, 194, 199
  clubbing of the fingers and, 155
  dullness to percussion of the chest
    and, 158
  easy bruising and, 112
  effects of, 203
  extremity signs and, 202, 297t
  family history and, 190–191, 193–
    195, 198–200
  fundus symptoms and, 196t
  gastrointestinal signs and, 194, 199
  general health of patient with, 193
  hair signs and, 199

Splenomegaly, *(continued)*
    hand symptoms and, 201, 195t
    head symptoms and, 191, 196t
    heart failure and, 217t
    history of patient with, 199
    jaundice and, 185
    laboratory studies and, 188–189,
        191–192, 202
    life situation and, 190–191, 195,
        199–200
    mental status and, 200
    mimicking by other diseases, 187
    musculoskeletal signs and, 194, 199
    neck symptoms and, 191, 201, 196t
    occupational hazards and, 200
    occupational history and, 195
    physical examination of patient
        with, 188, 195, 197, 200–202,
        195t, 196t, 197t
    pleural effusions and, 172–173
    precordial signs and, 201, 196t
    pulse measurements and, 195t
    rectal signs and, 202
    respiratory signs and, 194, 199
    scrotal signs and, 197t
    signs pathognomic of, 187
    signs suggestive of, 187–188
    skin symptoms and, 191, 193–194,
        199–200, 196t
    splenic notch and, 188
    thoracic signs and, 191, 201, 196t
    throat symptoms and, 199
    vital signs and, 200
    weight loss and, 19t

Vomiting,
    abdominal signs and, 66–71
    alcohol consumption and, 64t
    breast cancer patient, 68–69
    breast symptoms and, 65
    cardiovascular symptoms and, 64
    case of girl, 62, 65
    case of man, 65
    causes of, 58–62, 65, 69
    central nervous system symptoms
        and, 69, 63t
    chest pain and, 47–48
    diabetes mellitus and, 86t
    diagnostically significant
        characteristics of, 60–62
    drug addiction and, 64t
    effects of, 72–73
    extremity symptoms and, 67, 71
    family history and, 64t
    gastrointestinal symptoms and, 60,
        63t
    general appearance of patient, 67
    general health of patient, 64t
    genitourinary signs and, 65, 63t
    gastrointestinal symptoms and, 63t
    hand symptoms and, 70
    head signs and, 67, 70
    history of patient, 58–62, 66, 69–70,
        72–73, 64t
    hypertension and, 132
    hypotension and, 142
    jaundice and, 180–181, 186
    laboratory tests and, 68, 71–72
    life situation and, 64t
    medication history and, 65, 64t
    mental status and, 67, 70
    neck symptoms and, 71
    physical examination of patient, 66,
        70–73
    polyuria and, 77t
    rectal signs and, 67
    skin symptoms and, 68
    vital signs and, 67, 70

Weight loss,
    abdominal symptoms and, 14, 19t
    axillary lymph nodes and, 19t
    bacterial endocarditis and, 21–22
    breast signs and, 16–17, 19t
    cardiovascular signs and, 15
    case of man with, 8–9, 21–22
    causes of, 8–9
    cigarette use and, 18
    clubbing of the fingers and, 150
    confirmation of, 8
    depression and, 10–11
    diabetes mellitus as cause of, 85t
    extremity signs and, 19t
    eye signs and, 19t
    facial signs and, 19t
    family history of patient with, 17
    fundus signs and, 19t
    gastrointestinal symptoms and,
        9–10, 14
    general appearance of patient with,
        19t
    genital symptoms in woman
        showing, 16
    genitourinary signs in man showing,
        15
    geographic factors and, 18

Weight loss, *(continued)*
  hand symptoms and, 19t
  head symptoms and, 19t
  history of patient with, 17
  hypertension and, 135
  infectious diseases causing, 18–22
  life situation and, 17–18
  lymph nodes and, 19t
  malignant disease causing, 11–18
  medication history and, 18
  musculoskeletal signs and, 15–16
  neck signs and, 19t
  nervous system symptoms and, 16
  occupational factors and, 18
  physical examination of patient
    with, 8, 11–18, 21, 19t

  pleural effusion and, 167t
  polyuria and, 77t
  ptosis and, 225t
  rectal signs and, 19t
  respiratory symptoms and, 14
  scrotal signs and, 19t
  significance of, 7–8
  skin symptoms and, 16, 19t
  spinal signs and, 19t
  splenomegaly and, 192
  sputal examination and, 21, 22
  thoracic signs and, 19t
  tuberculosis as cause of, 20–21
  vomiting and, 79